中华五福

Designs of Chinese Blessings

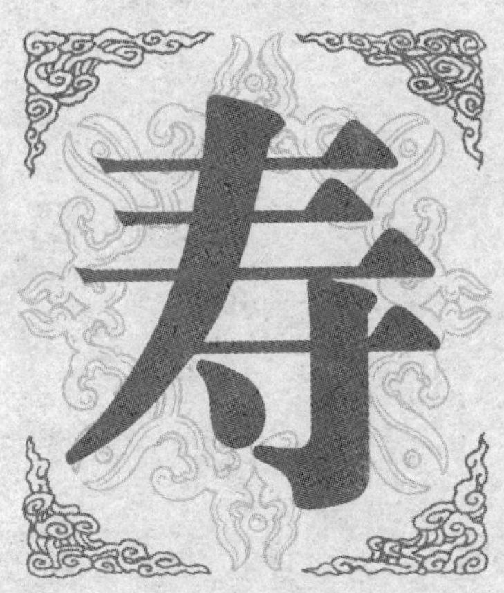

Longevity

主　编／黄全信
副主编／黄 迎　李 进
编　委／吴曼丽　王玉智　陈 惠　龚 卓
林美倩　楚晓彬　崔 婷　叶乐萌
翻　译／李迎春

华语教学出版社
SINOLINGUA

First Edition 2003

ISBN 7-80052-890-1

Published by Sinolingua
24 Baiwanzhuang Road, Beijing 100037, China
Tel: (86) 10-68995871/68326333
Fax: (86) 10-68326333
E-mail: hyjx @263.net
Printed by Beijing Foreign Languages Printing House
Distributed by China International
Book Trading Corporation
35 Chegongzhuang Xilu, P.O.Box 399
Beijing 100044, China

Printed in the People's Republic of China

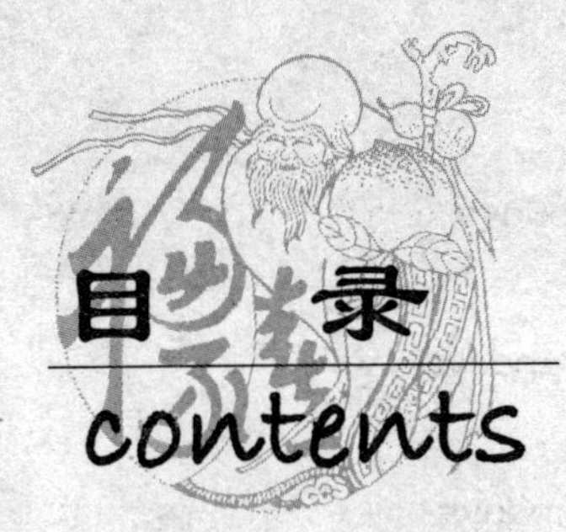

目录

contents

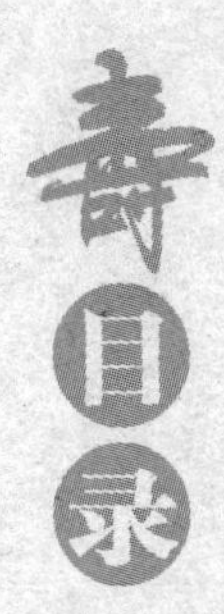

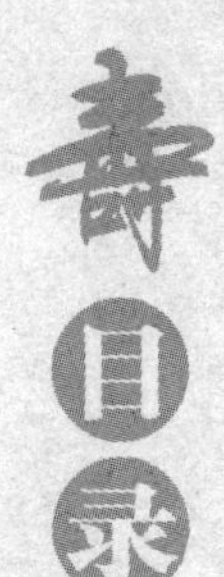

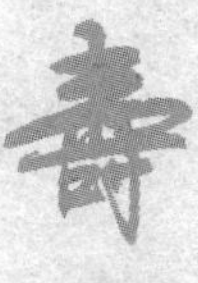

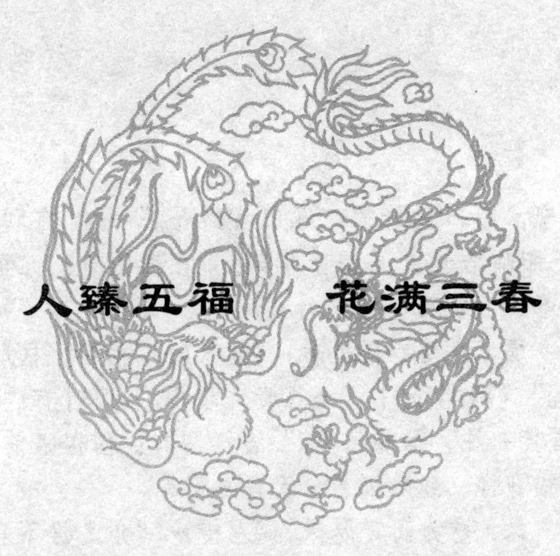

人臻五福　花满三春

吉祥一词，始见于《易经》："吉事有祥。"《左传》有："是何祥也？吉祥焉在？"《庄子》则有："虚室生日，吉祥止止。"《注疏》云："吉者，福善之事；祥者，嘉庆之征。"

吉祥二字，在甲骨文中被写作"吉羊"。上古人过着游牧生活，羊肥大成群是很"吉祥"的事，在古器物的铭文中多有"吉羊"。《说文》云："羊，祥也。"

吉祥，是美好、幸运的形象；吉祥，是人类最迷人的主题。艺术，最终都是把理想形象化；吉祥图，是中华吉祥文化最璀璨的明珠。旧时有联："善果皆欢喜，香云普吉祥。"吉祥图有：吉祥如意、五福吉祥等。

五福，是吉祥的具体。福、禄、寿、喜、财，在民间被称为五福；福星、禄星、寿星、喜神、财神，在仙界被尊为五福神。五福最早见于《尚书》："五福：一曰寿，二曰富，三曰康宁，四曰攸好德，五曰考终命。”旧时有联：“三阳临吉地，五福萃华门。”吉祥图有：五福捧寿、三多五福等。

福，意为幸福美满。《老子》：“福兮，祸所伏。”《韩非子》：“全富贵之谓福。”旧时有联：“香焚一炷，福赐三多。”吉祥图有：福在眼前、纳福迎祥、翘盼福音、天官赐福等。

禄，意为高官厚禄。《左传》：“介之推不言禄，禄亦弗及。”《汉书》：“身宠而载高位，家温而食厚禄。”旧时有联：“同科十进士，庆榜三名元。”吉祥图有：禄位高升、福禄寿禧、天赐禄爵、加官进禄等。

寿，意为健康长寿。《庄子》：“人，上寿百岁，中寿八十，下寿六十。”《诗经》：“如南山之寿，不骞不崩。”旧时有联：“同臻寿域，共跻春台。”吉祥图有：寿星高照、鹤寿千年、富贵寿考、蟠桃献寿等。

喜，意为欢乐喜庆。《国语》：“固庆其喜而吊其忧。”韦昭注：“喜犹福也。”旧时有联：“笑到几时方合口，坐来无日不开怀。”吉祥图有：喜上眉梢、双喜临门、端阳喜庆、皆大欢喜等。

财，意为发财富有。《荀子》：“务本节用财无极。”旧时有联：“生意兴隆通四海，财源茂盛达三江。”吉祥图有：财源滚滚、招财进宝、喜交财运、升官发财等。

吉祥图，不仅有“五福”之内涵，而且是

绘画艺术和语言艺术的珠联璧合。在绘画上，体现了中国画主要的表现手段——线的魅力，给人以美感，令人赏心悦目。吉祥图虽多出自民间画工之手，却多有顾恺之“春蚕吐丝”之韵，曹仲达“曹衣出水”之美，吴道子“吴带当风”之妙；在语言上，通俗和普及了古代文化，吉祥图多配有一句浓缩成四个字的吉语祥词，给人以吉祥，令人心驰神往。

《中华五福吉祥图典》，汇集了我数代家传和几十年收藏的精品吉祥图，可谓美不胜收。其中既有明之典雅，又有清之华丽；既有皇家之富贵，又有民间之纯朴；既有北方之粗犷，又有南方之秀美……按五福全书分成福、禄、寿、喜、财五集，每集吉祥图 119 幅，共 595 幅。除同类图案外，均按笔画顺序编排。基本包括了中国传统吉祥图的各个方面，并对每幅图作了考证和诠释，使之图文并茂，相得益彰。

五福人人喜，吉祥家家乐。吉祥图是中国的，也是世界的，故以汉英对照出版。《中华五福吉祥图典》会给您带来吉祥，给您全家带来幸福。

黄全信于佩实斋

2003 年 1 月 1 日

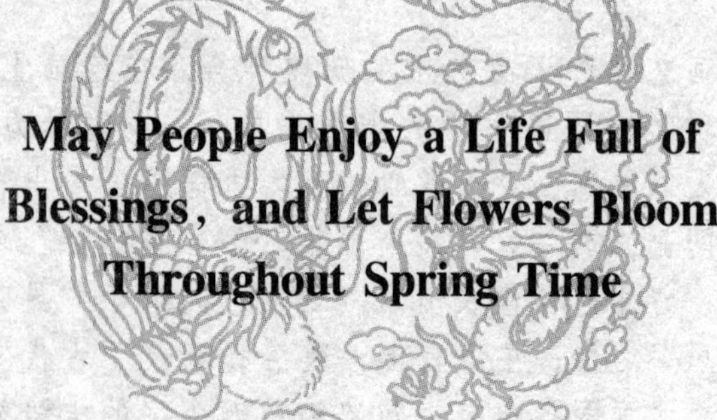

May People Enjoy a Life Full of Blessings, and Let Flowers Bloom Throughout Spring Time

The word jixiang (meaning lucky, propitious, or auspicious) is mentioned in Chinese ancient books and writings as early as in the Zhou Dynasty.

The word jixiang was written as jiyang (lucky sheep) on oracle bones. To the ancient Chinese, who led a nomadic life, large herds of well-fed sheep were auspicious things, and the word jiyang also appeared in engravings on ancient utensils.

To have good luck is mankind's eternal desire. While art records man's ideals, good luck pictures are the most brilliant part of the Chinese good luck culture. An old couplet says that kindness leads to happiness and good luck. Typical good luck pictures are: good luck and heart's content, good luck with five blessings, etc.

The five blessings – good fortune, high salary and a good career, longevity, happiness, and wealth – are the concrete forms of good luck , and there are five

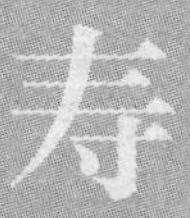

kinds of gods presiding over these blessings. The five blessings as they are first mentioned in Chinese literature are not quite the same as the five which are talked about today, though they are quite similar. An old couplet says that as the land of good luck bathes in the Sun, a prosperous family is granted all the blessings. Typical good luck pictures are: long-term enjoyment of all five blessings, more blessings, etc.

Good fortune means happiness and complete satisfaction. Ancient Chinese philosophers, including Lao Zi, all commented on the notion of good fortune. An old couplet says to burn incense to beg for more blessings. Good luck pictures in this theme include good fortune for today, blessings from above, etc.

High salary means handsome salaries at prestigious posts. In old times, Chinese attached great significance to academic excellence, which led in turn to high positions in government. An old couplet says may you distinguish yourselves in the royal examinations and rank at the top of the list. Good luck pictures in this theme used in this book include big improvements in salary and post, salary and position bestowed from heaven, etc.

Longevity refers to good health and a long life. As Zhuangzhou said, and the *Book of Songs* records, longevity is the universal wish of mankind. As wished in an old couplet, to grow to a long life together is a joyful experience . This book has the following good luck pic -

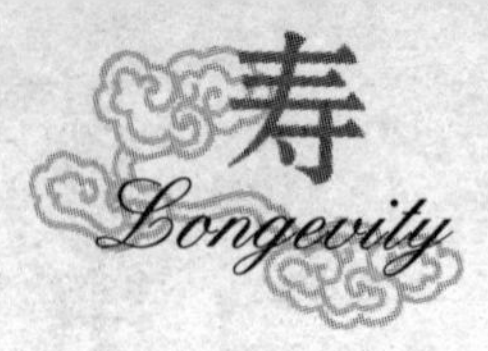

tures concerning longevity: high above shines the star of longevity, live to be 1, 000 years with white hair, and offer the flat peach to wish for longevity, etc.

Happiness refers to happy events and celebrations. Happy events should be celebrated, while those with worries should be consoled according to ancient Chinese literature. An old Chinese couplet says, why not keep on laughing as all days are filled with happiness. Good luck pictures on this theme included in this book include double happiness visits at the door, all's well that ends well, etc.

Wealth means getting rich and having plentiful things. Ancient Chinese believed that the secret to endless wealth is to be down-to-earth and prudent. Illustrating the concept of wealth is an old couplet: a prosperous business deals with people from all corners of the world, and wealth rolls in from afar. Typical good luck pictures of this type include in comes wealth, get rich and win high positions, etc.

Good luck pictures not only incorporate the five blessings but the art of painting and language as well. The beautiful lines of these pictures, done in the style of traditional Chinese painting, provide the viewers with artistic enjoyment which is pleasing to the eyes and heart. Though mostly the work of folk artists, they exhibit a level of craftsmanship worthy of the great and famous masters. The language adopted in these pictures serves to popularize ancient culture, and the four-character good luck phrase accompanying almost every picture depicts an attractive scene.

Designs of Chinese Blessings is a compilation of special good luck pictures passed down in my family for several generations as well those which I have been collecting for dozens of years. Their beauty is beyond description. They combine the elegance of the Ming Dynasty and the magnificence of the Qing Dynasty, the nobility of the royal family and the modesty of the common people, the boldness of the north and the delicacy of the south. The book consists of five sections: good fortune, high salary and a good career, longevity, happiness, and wealth. With 119 pictures in each section, the whole book contains 595 pictures and is a complete representation of the various aspects of traditional Chinese good luck pictures. On top of this, research has been done on each picture, and the interpretations complement the visuals nicely.

As the five blessings are the aspiration of each individual, good luck delights all households. The good luck pictures originated in China and their good message should benefit all people of this world. May the *Designs of Chinese Blessings* bring good luck to your life and happiness to your family.

Huang Quanxin

Jan.1, 2003

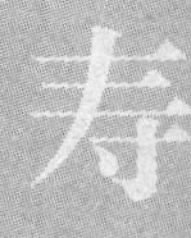

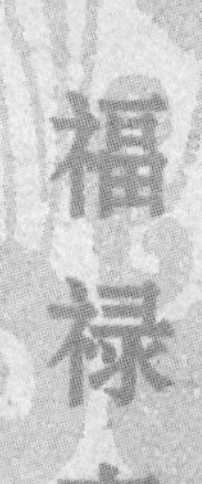

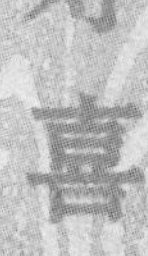

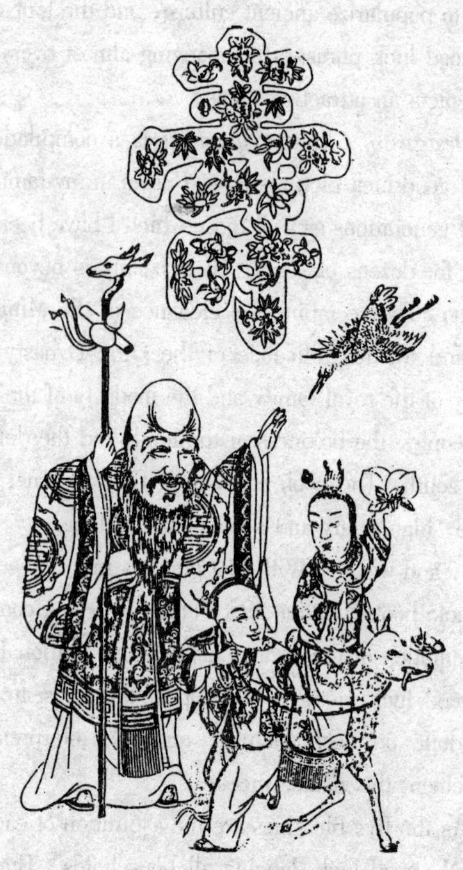

人歌上寿

Celebrating Longevity

《庄子》：“人，上寿百岁，中寿八十，下寿六十。”五福唯寿为重，人活七十古来稀，人至上寿乃大吉。寿联云：“君子有诗歌偕老，上寿自古称大齐。”年轻人庆生辰，只能称“过生日”，50或60岁以上者方可称“庆寿”。

Ancient Chinese considered the age of 100 supreme longevity, the age of 80 medium longevity, and the age of 60 low longevity. Of the five blessings, longevity is the most important of all. As the age 70 was a rarity in old times, one is bestowed with even better fortune if one reaches the age of 100. A birthday celebration couplet reads: “As gentlemen mature in age with songs, he who is 100 years old has great achievements”. While young people hold birthday parties, only those aged 50 or 60 and above celebrate longevity.

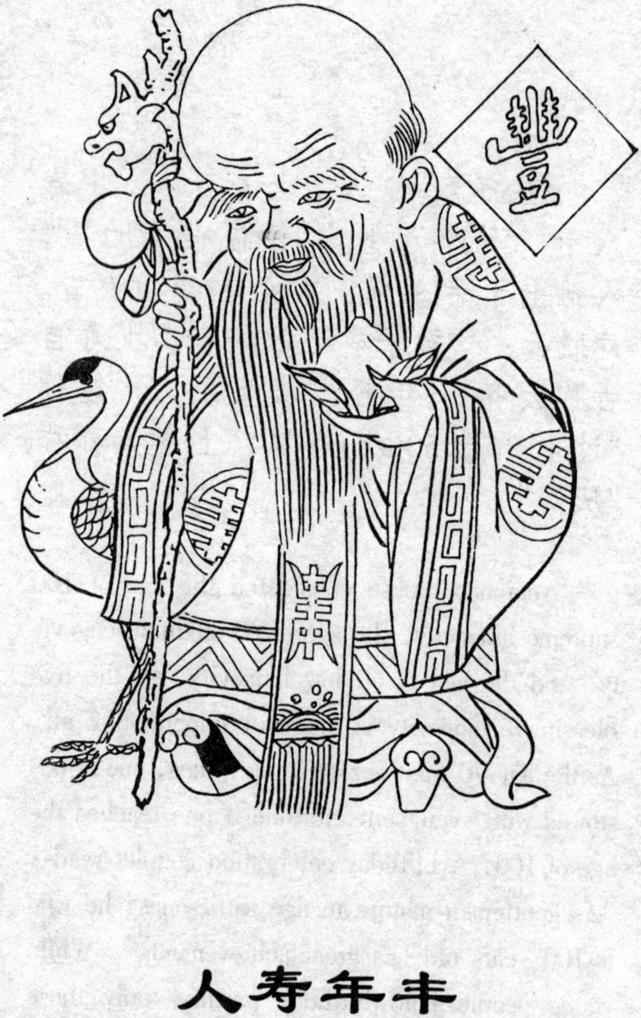

人寿年丰

Longevity to man with a havest year

《诗经》："如南山之寿，不骞不崩。"人以寿为本，民以食为天。旧时有春联："人人寿比南山，年年丰衣足食。"横披为："人寿年丰"。人寿，仁者长寿；年丰，勤者年丰。长寿，是一生最大的幸福；丰收，是一年最大的企盼。

The *Book of Songs* says "May people reach a very senior age and stay healthy as the mountains". Food and longevity are both basic concerns of the people. A spring couplet from the past goes "May everyone live a long time like the enduring mountains and let there be adequate clothing and food" and the horizontal scroll reads "Longevity to man and harvest every year". Longevity, the greatest happiness in life, is associated with kindness; harvest, expected in earnest through the year, is a reward to the industrious.

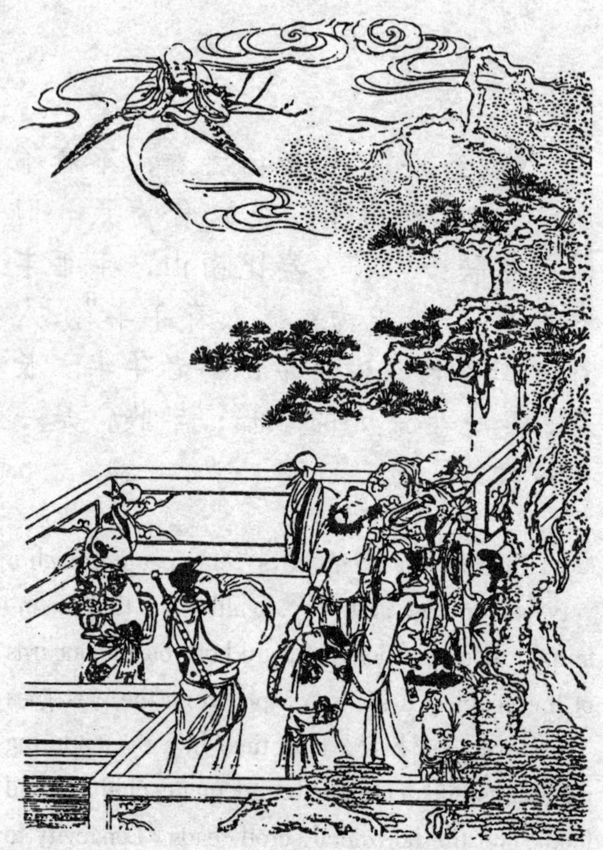

八仙仰寿

The eight immortals look up to offer birthday peaches and toasts

《神异记》：西王母每逢蟠桃成熟的三月初三，便大摆寿宴，邀请各路神仙赴蟠桃盛会，为她祝寿。王母乘凤于云间，下有八仙献桃献酒，称为仰寿。民间祝贺女寿往往画王母娘娘，而祝贺男寿则画寿星，以求"年年如意，岁岁平安"。

Ancient Chinese stories about the gods tell us that the Queen Mother of the West would set up a grand feast to celebrate her birthday on March 3rd, an occasion coinciding with the harvest season of flat peaches. Immortals of different schools are invited to attend the grand gathering to congratulate her. As the Queen Mother rides on a phoenix in the clouds, the eight immortals would offer her peaches and wine from below. In folk practices, the Queen Mother appears on birthday congratulation pictures where the celebration is for a woman while the god of longevity appears where the celebration is for a man.

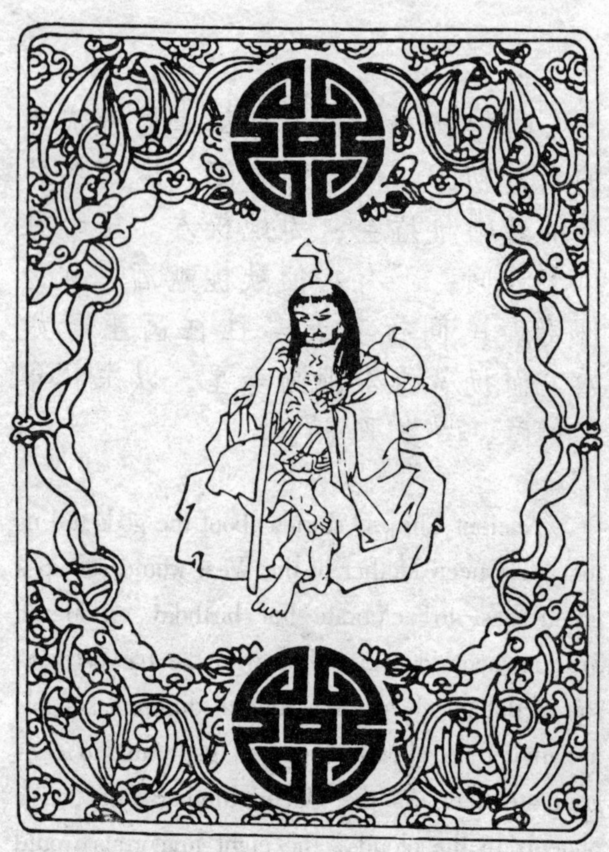

李铁拐庆寿

Tieguai Li congratulates birthdays

李铁拐在八仙中资历最深，姓李，因腿跛拄一根铁拐杖，故名铁拐李。一说他是隋朝人，一说他是老子的学生。他有一只内装灵丹妙药的宝葫芦，为人治病去灾，故民间也把他视为医药行业神，并视他为狗皮膏药的发明者。

Tieguai Li is the most senior of the eight immortals. His family name is Li and he rode on an iron stick to support his lame leg, hence the title Tie (iron) Guai (stick) Li. There are two versions of his origin: one says that he was from the Sui Dynasty and the other says that he was a student of Laozi of Zhou. He had a treasure bottle gourd with magic medicine in it and he would cure people suffering from diseases, which was why common people also saw him as the god of medicine and regarded him as the inventor of quack medicine.

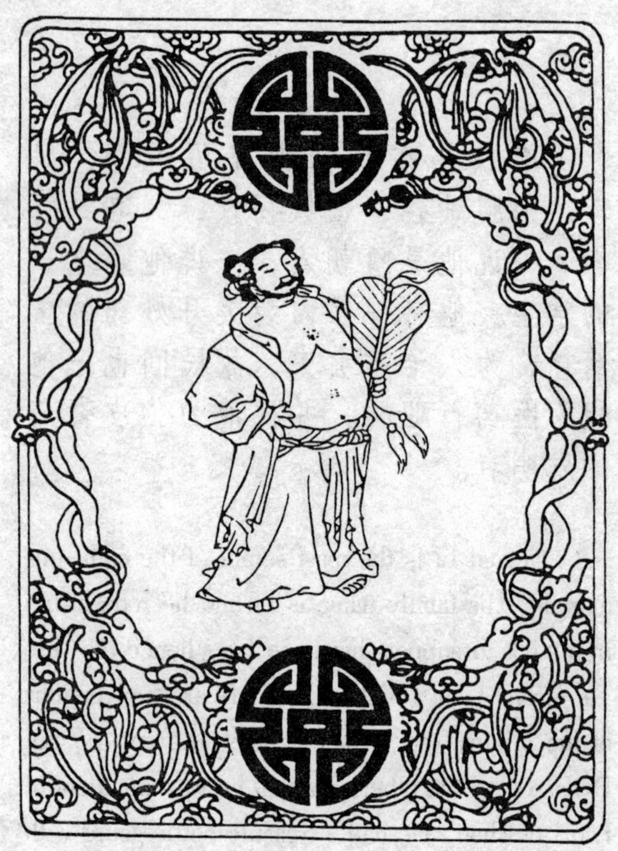

钟离权庆寿

Zhongli Quan congratulates birthdays

钟离权，姓钟离，名权。相传为汉朝人，故又称汉钟离。传说钟离权的父亲征讨匈奴有功，被封为汉燕台侯。他也荫封为将，因吃败仗，才学道成仙。他头梳两个丫髻，袒胸露腹，手拿棕扇，神态闲散，被称为天下第一闲散之人。

It is said that Zhongli (the family name) Quan was from the Han Dynasty which explains why he is also called Han Zhongli. Legend says that his father made great achievements in a military expedition against the Hsiung-Nu and was bestowed a high position. Zhongli Quan, too, was offered the post of general but encountered defeats. So he turned to study Taoism and became an immortal. He had two braids on his head and exposed his chest and belly. With a palm fan in his hand and looking very relaxed, Han Zhongli was the very expression of idleness.

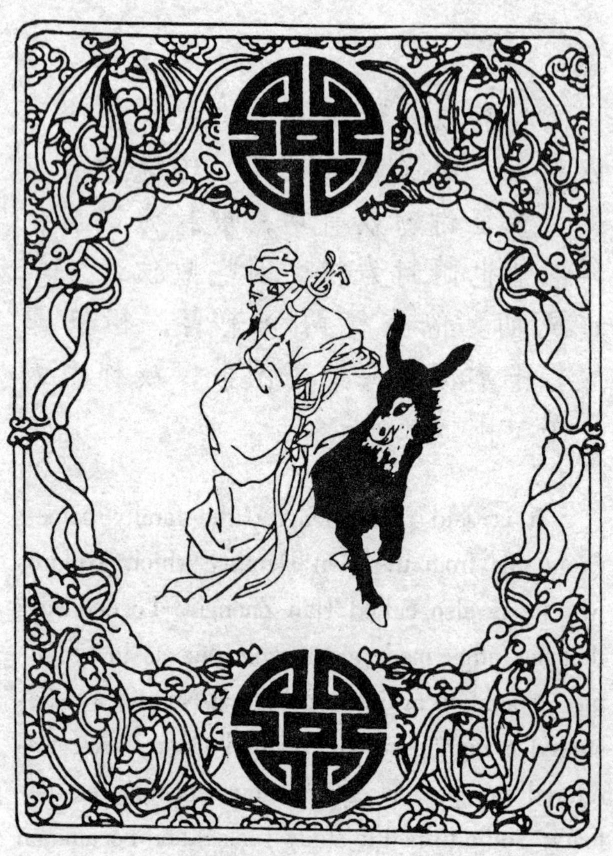

张果老庆寿

Zhang Guolao congratulates birthdays

张果老，原名张果，唐朝进士。他总以老人的面目出现，声称年逾数百岁，故称张果老。张果老有两件宝，一是他手中的鱼鼓，另一是他坐下的毛驴，此驴可日行万里。张果老玩世不恭，倒骑毛驴。另说张果老是白蝙蝠所化。

Zhang Guolao's original name is Zhang Guo and he was a successful candidate in the highest imperial examinations of the Tang Dynasty. He always appeared as an old person and claimed himself to be over 100 years old, hence the title Zhang Guolao (lao meaning old). He had two treasures – a wooden fish and a short donkey which could travel for 10,000 li a day. Zhang Guolao practiced Bohemianism – he rode his donkey with his back facing front. Another version of his origin is that he was made man from a white bat.

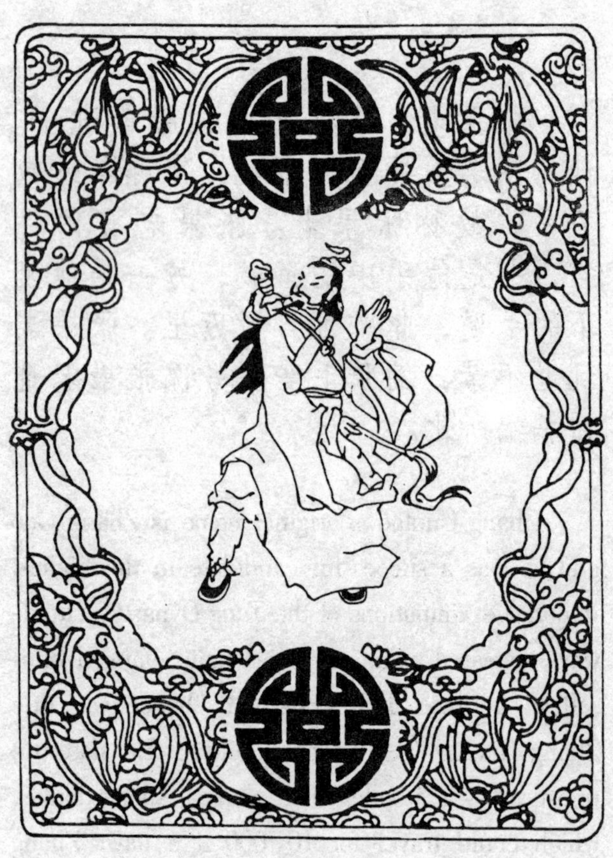

吕洞宾庆寿

Lü Dongbin congratulates birthdays

吕洞宾在八仙中名气最大，各地均有吕祖庙。吕洞宾原名吕宾，唐朝人，屡试不第，后被钟离权点化得道，还得火龙真人的“遁天剑法”。元、明时，被朝廷封为纯阳帝君，还被全真道教奉为纯阳祖师，为道教的三祖之一。

Lü Dongbin is the most reputed of the eight immortals and temples after him have been built in all places. Originally under the name of Lü Bin, Lü Dongbin lived in the Tang Dynasty. After many failures in the royal examinations, he was enlightened by Zhongli Han and mastered the skills of sword playing. During the Yuan and Ming Dynasties, the emperor bestowed on him the title of supreme master. He is also worshipped as one of the three founders of Taoism.

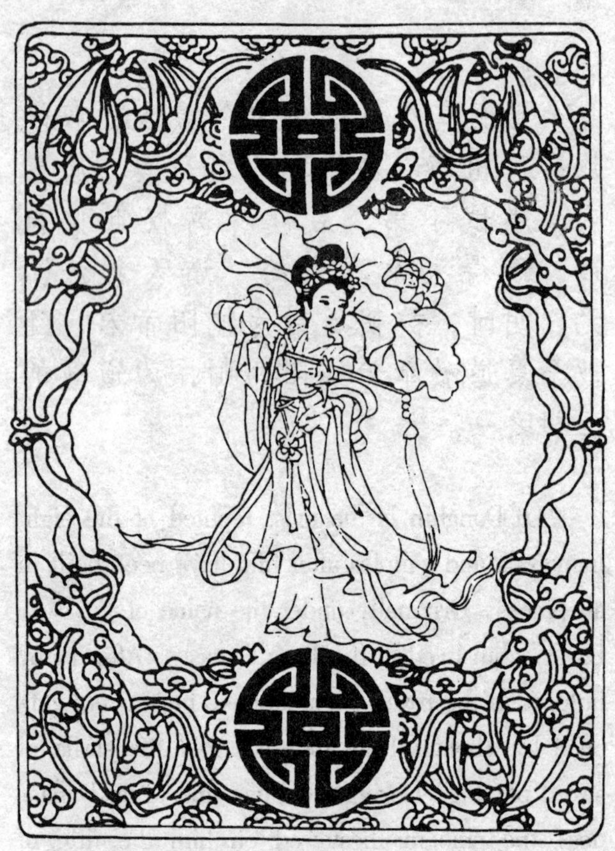

何仙姑庆寿

He Xiangu congratulates birthdays

何仙姑是八仙中唯一的女性。传说她是唐代岭南人，名琼。她出生时有紫云绕室，顶有六毫。十三岁时，山中遇道士赠桃成仙，终身不嫁。往来山间，身轻如飞。何仙姑为一美貌少女形象，手执荷花，有“手执荷花不染尘”之誉。

He Xiangu is the only woman of the eight immortals. It is said that she was from south China in the Tang Dynasty. At the time of her birth, purple clouds surrounded the house. At the age of 13, she met a Taoist priest in the mountain and received a peach. She became a fairy and vowed never to get married in her life. As she traveled between the mountains, her movements were so light that she seemed to be flying. The image of He Xiangu is a pretty young girl holding a lotus, a plant unspoiled though rooted in mud.

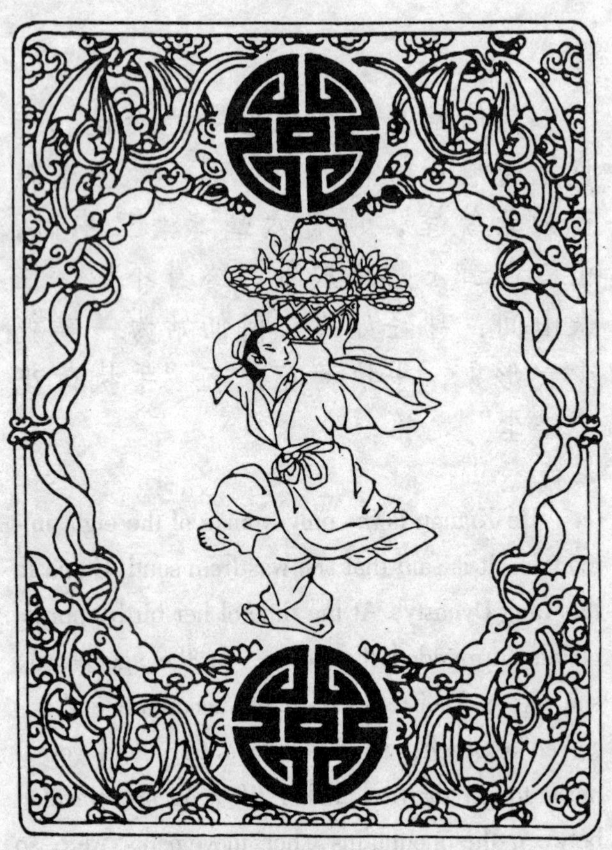

蓝采和庆寿

Lan Caihe congratulates birthdays

蓝采和，不知何许人也。经常是衣衫褴褛，腰系宽木带，一脚着靴，一脚赤裸，夏日衫内加絮，冬天卧于雪中。常手执三尺大板，行乞街头，老少皆随看之，为其机敏谐谑倾倒。他把讨来的钱用长绳串起，沿街抛撒，周济穷人。

Lan Caihe's origin is unknown. He often appeared ragged with a wide wooden belt in the waist with one bare foot. In summer time, he had cotton padded clothes and in winter, he laid on snow. He held a three-foot long board to beg on the streets and crowds of people, old and young, would follow him to get entertained by his smartness and humor. He put the coins he begged in a long string and scatter them along the streets to aid the poor.

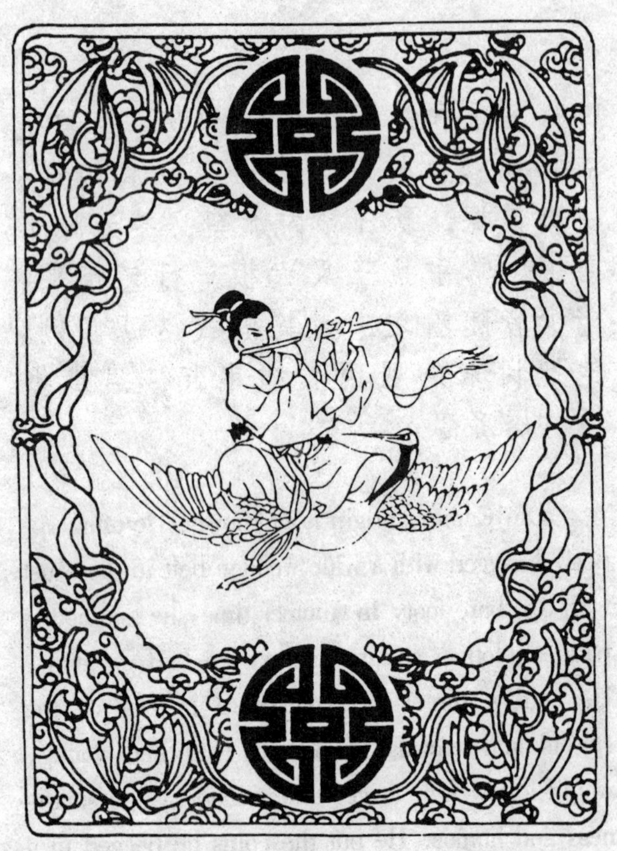

韩湘子庆寿

Han Xiangzi congratulates birthdays

相传汉丞相安抚有个美貌的女儿灵灵，皇帝欲把她给侄儿当媳妇，安抚不允，汉皇怒罢安抚。灵灵郁闷而死变为白鹤，经钟离权、吕洞宾点化，投生为韩会之子，名湘子，由叔父唐代大文豪韩愈养育成人，又经点化终成正果。

It is said that An Fu, a prime minister from the Han Dynasty had a beautiful daughter named Lingling and the emperor intended to marry her to his nephew. An Fu disallowed this and the angered emperor removed An Fu from his post. Lingling was so depressed that she died and turned into a white crane. Enlightened by Zhongli Quan and Lü Dongbin, the crane reincarnated in the body of the son of Han Hui under the name Xiangzi. Raised up by his uncle Han Yu, the literary giant of the Tang Dynasty, he finally reached the spiritual state of an immortal.

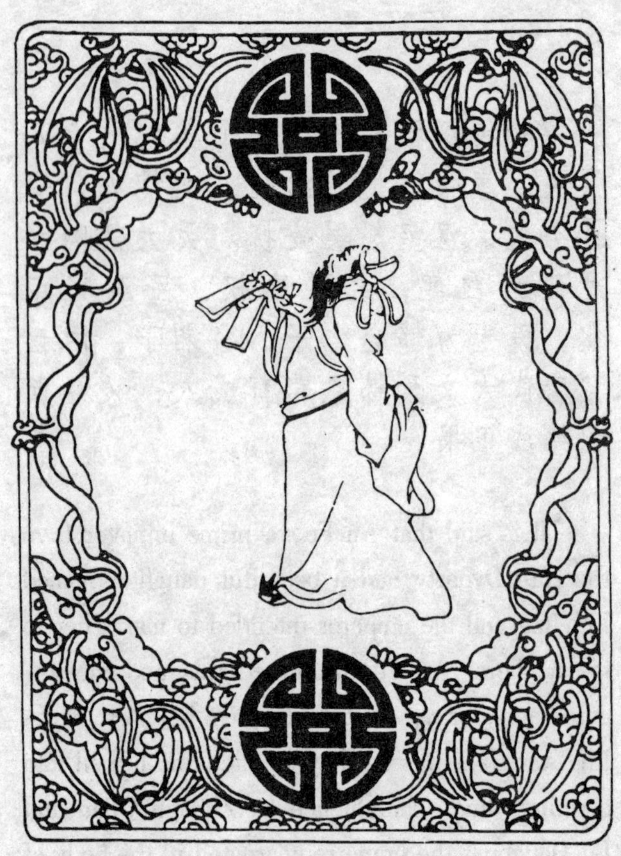

曹国舅庆寿

Cao Guojiu congratulates birthdays

曹国舅名友，是宋仁宗曹皇后的大弟，因此称为国舅。他的弟弟依仗姐姐的权势作恶，曹友深以为耻，于是把家产散发穷人，隐居山中。后经钟离权、吕洞宾点化成道。曹国舅是八仙中唯一的高官，总是手拿笏板，一身官服。

Cao Guojiu was the eldest younger brother of the empress of Song Ren Zong. His younger brother indulged himself in evil deeds on reliance of his special status as the brother of the empress and Cao Guojiu was very ashamed of this. He scattered his household properties among the poor and led a reclusive life in the mountains. Enlightened by Zhongli Quan and Lü Dongbin, he became an immortal. The only high official of the eight immortals, Cao Guojiu always appeared in pictures in official costumes with a tablet in his hand.

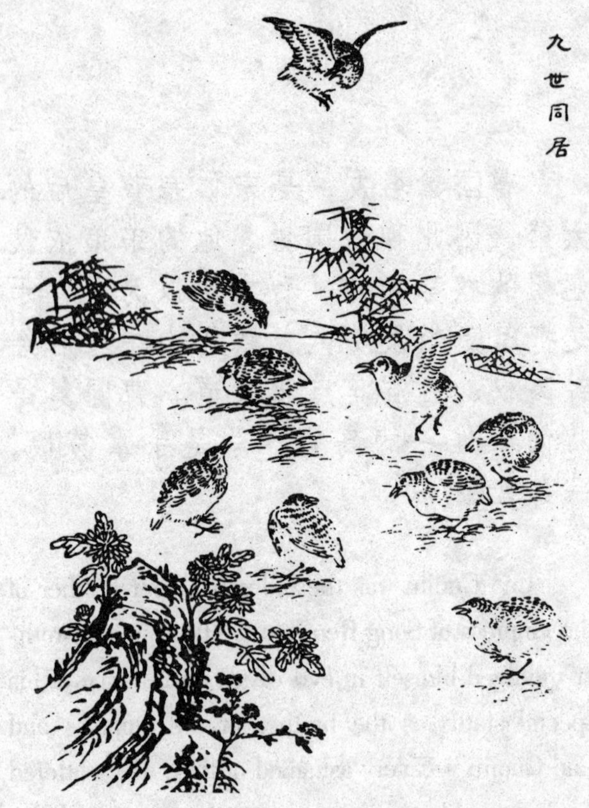

九世同居

Nine generations under the same roof

《唐书·孝友传序》："张公艺，九世同居，高宗有事泰山，临幸其居，问本末，书'忍'字百余以对，天子为流涕，赐缣帛而去。"四世同堂已为不易，九世同居更是难得。后人常以九世同居示家庭和睦，多以九只鹌鹑偕菊喻之。

A book on the history of the Tang Dynasty records that there were nine generations of people living in the same house in Zhang Gongyi's family. The first emperor of Tang visited him and asked how he could handle all these. Zhang wrote the character "tolerance" for over 100 times and the emperor was moved to tears. Four generations of people living in the same house is not a common thing and nine generations is even more difficult to come by. The expression is later cited as a reference to family harmony and nine quails picking chrysanthemums (a pun with "living" in Chinese) is the typical picture for it.

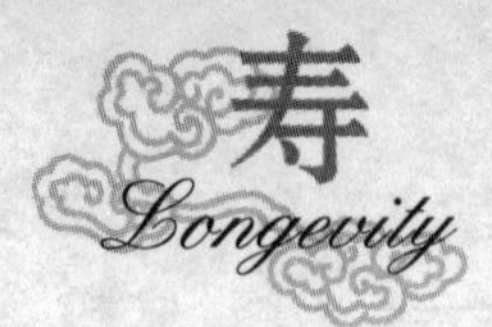

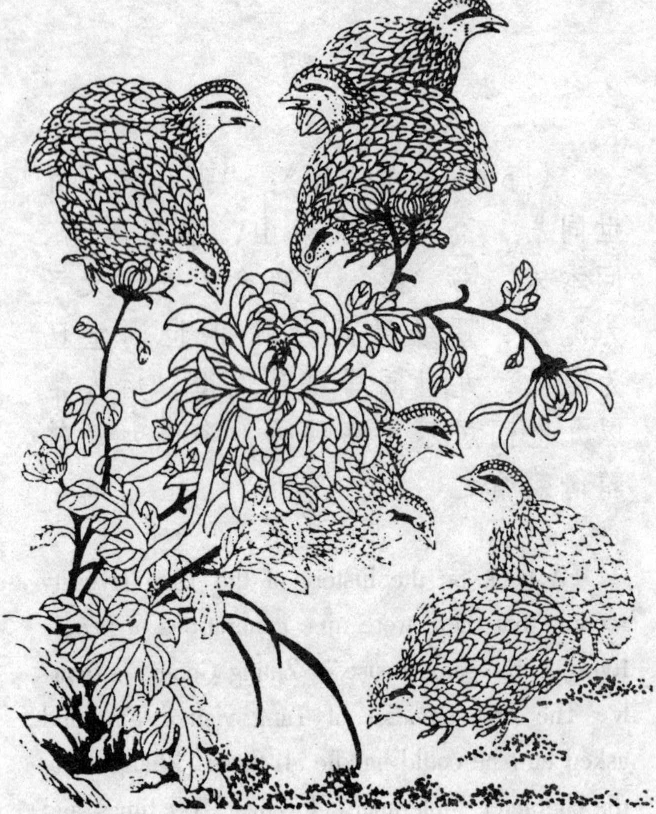

九世同居

Nine generations under the same roof

图中“九只”鹌鹑与“九世”谐音，“同”株之“菊”与“同居”谐音，合为“九世同居”。讲的是唐代寿张人张公艺，九世同居。唐高宗封泰山时，去过他家，问他如何能九世同居，张公艺写了一百个忍字，皇帝感动赐他缣帛。

The nine quails and the chrysanthemums in the picture stand for nine generations under the same roof (due to similarity in pronunciation). The story is about Zhang Gongyi in the Tang Dynasty and the nine generations of people in his family. The first emperor of Tang visited him and asked how he could handle all these. Zhang wrote the character "tolerance" for over 100 times and the emperor, moved to tears, gave him some silk to show his respect.

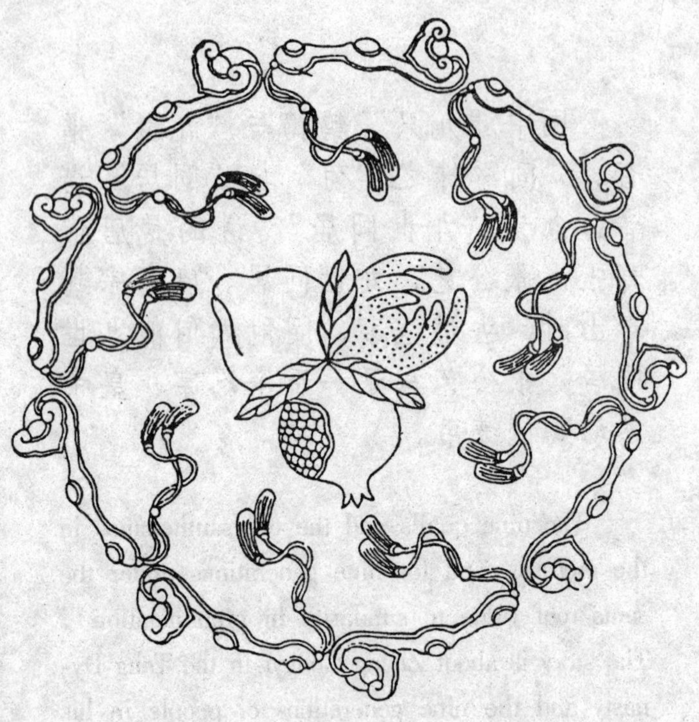

三多九如

Plentiful blessings

三多，为多福、多寿、多子。九如见《诗·小雅·天保》：“如山如阜，如冈如陵，如川之方至，以莫不增……如月之恒，如日之升，如南山之寿，不骞不崩，如松柏之茂，无不尔或承。”文中连用九个如字，以赞颂福寿绵长。

The Chinese cherish good fortune, longevity, and many children. Ancient Chinese men of letters used nine comparisons to describe the beauty and boundlessness of good fortune and longevity. These nine comparisons are: like mountains and mounds, like mounts and uninterrupted stretches of hills, like rivers flowing over from afar, like the eternal moon, like the rising sun, like Mount Zhongnanshan, and like exuberant pines and cypresses.

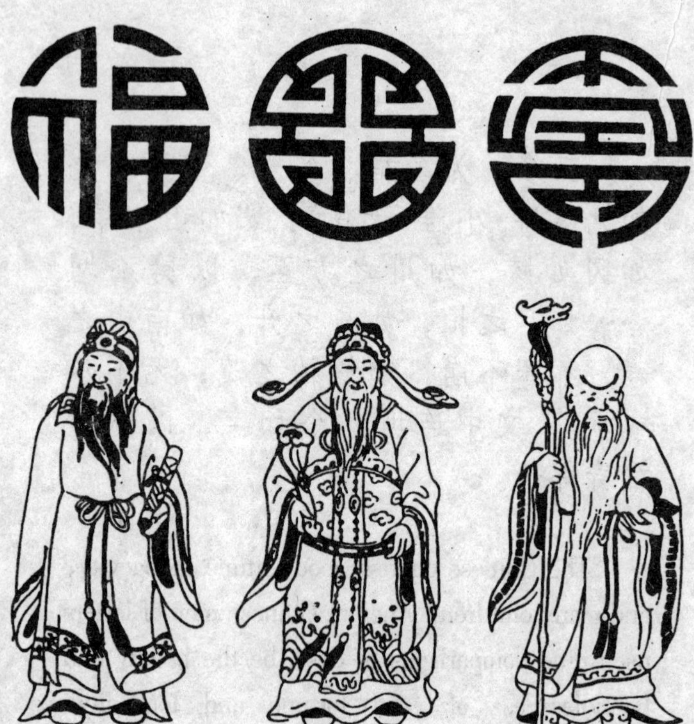

三星图

Picture of the three gods

三星，指福、禄、寿三星。即吏部天官福星，员外郎禄星，南极老人寿星。福星，头戴官冠，身着官服，手执朝笏或如意。禄星，为员外打扮，多怀抱婴儿。寿星，高额长须，一手执杖、一手捧桃。三星上方有福、禄、寿，三个园形篆字。

The three gods here refer to the gods of good fortune, salary, and longevity. The god of good fortune wears an official hat and costume with a tablet or *ruyi* in his hand, the god of salary is dressed like a ministry councilor with usually a baby in his arms, and the god of longevity has a large forehead and long beard with a walking stick in one hand and a peach in the other. Above the three stars are three round-shaped seal scripts for good fortune, salary and position, and longevity.

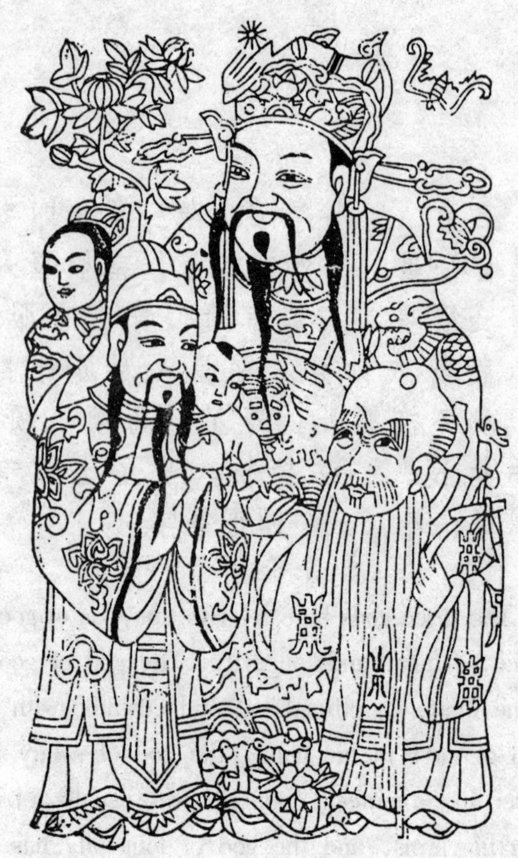

三星高照

High above shine the three stars

在福、禄、寿、喜、财五福中，福、禄、寿三星一起出现的吉祥图最多，意为“三星高照”。“三星高照”也称之为“三星在户”、“三星临门”、“三星图”、“福禄寿三星”等。有“三星高照”，必“五福临门”，是大吉。

Of all the good luck pictures, the three representations of good fortune, salary and position, and longevity appearing together are the most commonly seen. The picture of “high above shine the three stars” are also called “the three stars in the hall”, “the three stars at the doorstep”, etc. Where the three stars visit, the five blessings surely reside with the family.

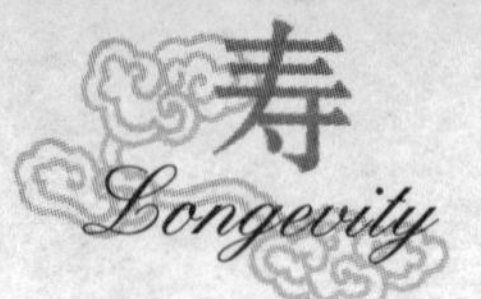

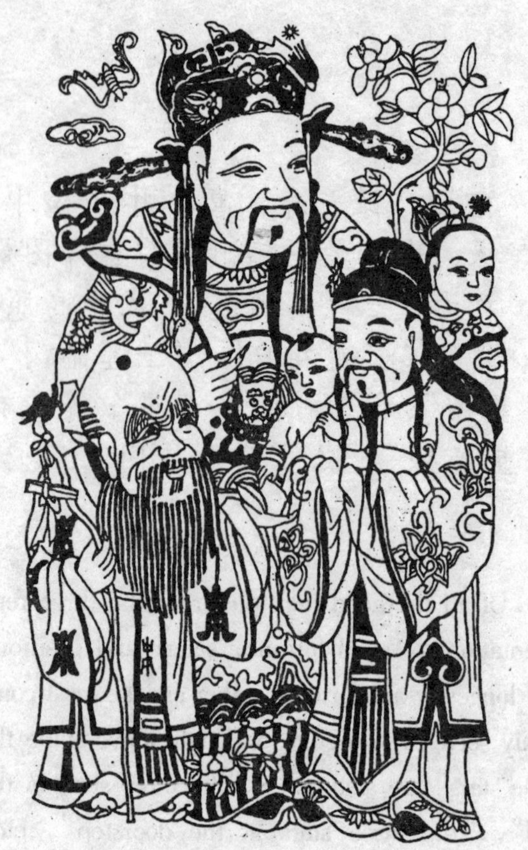

三星高照

High above shine the three stars

《礼记·中庸》："日月所照。"旧时有句："天上日月星，人间福禄寿。"福，为"五福"之总；禄，即俸禄，钱财，是人们生活的基础，旧时称"没什么别没钱"。寿，为"五福"之首。我国自古就有星象崇拜，故把福、禄、寿称"三星"。

Ancient Chinese worshipped the sun, the moon, and other stars in the sky. Therefore, the gods over good fortune, salary, and longevity are called the three stars. Good fortune summarizes the five blessings, salary stands for money that people depend on in life, and longevity is the first of the five blessings.

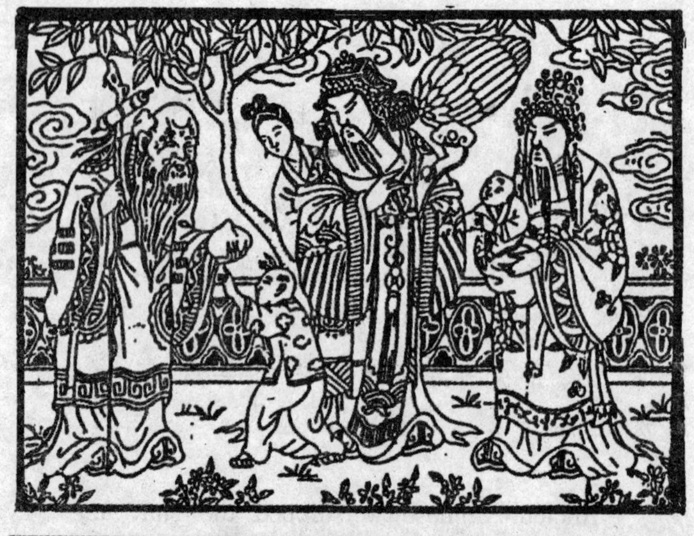

三星在户

The three stars in the hall

“三星”是福、禄、寿三星的简称，“在户”指在堂上。旧时习俗，每到春节的时候，人们总盼着三位吉星照临，以企新的一年生活幸福。有的在吉祥图中还配以吉词祥语，如：“三星在户，福寿绵长。”“三星在户，五福临门”。

The three stars preside over good fortune, salary, and longevity of the family. Under old customs, people would put up pictures of the three stars to welcome their arrival and blessing for the new year during the Spring Festival. There are couplets which go with these good luck pictures such as "long and lasting good fortune and longevity as the three star shine above".

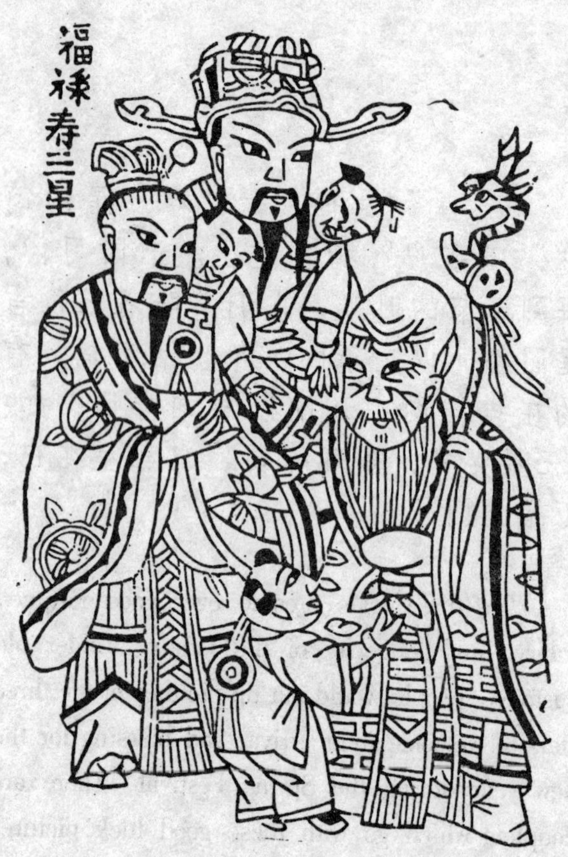

福禄寿三星

The three stars of good fortune, salary, and longevity

“福”如东海，“禄”位高升，“寿”比南山，每个都是大福。但“福善之事”多多宜善，故吉祥图中多把福、禄、寿三星合在一起，以求更大的福分，更多的吉祥。在吉祥图中，也有把其中二者集为一图的，如：“福寿无极”、“寿天百禄”等。

May good fortune abounds like the east sea, salary and position keep rising, and longevity last like the mountains. Each of the three is a great blessing in itself yet the aspiration for more blessings is limitless. Hence the three stars of good fortune, salary, and longevity are often put together in good luck pictures. Some good luck pictures have combinations of two of the three blessings.

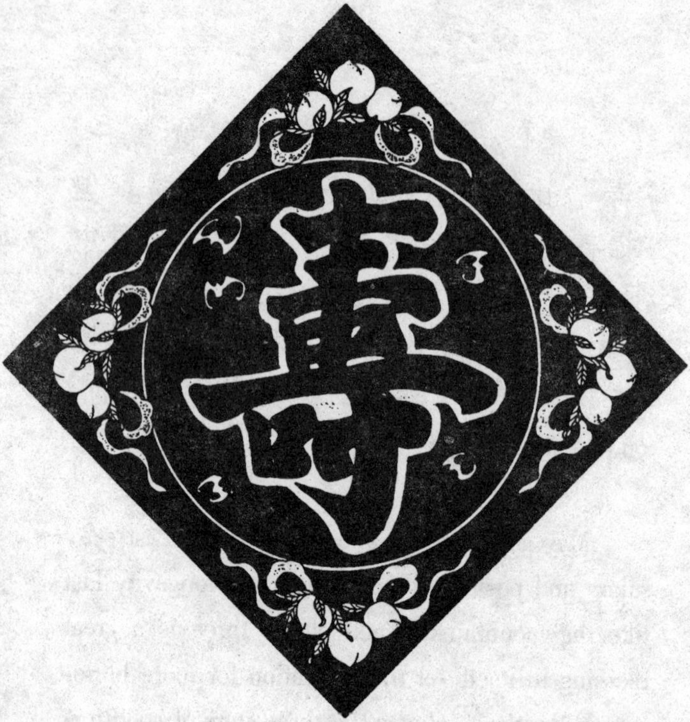

大寿之福

The good fortune of longevity

中国民间五福中有寿，三多中有寿，可见寿在人们心目中所占的位置。五福中寿居其首，五福捧寿寿居中心，大寿乃人之首福、大福。图中尚有“五福捧寿”、“蟠桃献寿”之意。长寿安康、永享天年是人类共同的美好愿望。

Longevity is among the five blessings in Chinese culture and a top priority in the minds of people. Longevity being the first and most essential of the five blessings, is sought after by all people. The picture also conveys messages like "longevity above all blessings", and "present flat peaches and wish for longevity". It is the universal aspiration of all people to enjoy a healthy long life.

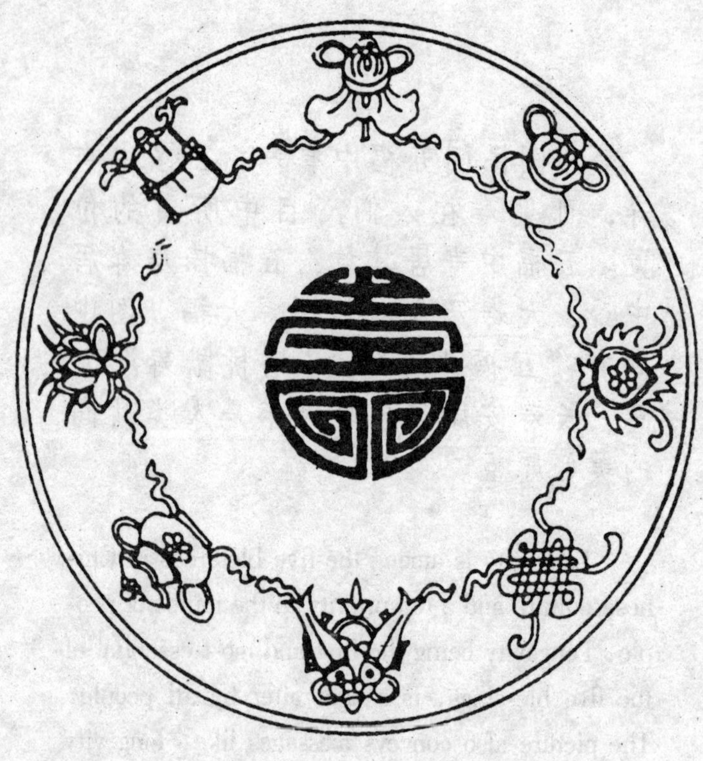

万寿八宝

The eight magic objects and longevity

佛教自汉代传入中国以来，佛教的法物也都成为了吉祥之物。八宝指：法螺、法轮、宝伞、白盖、莲花、宝瓶、金鱼、盘长。且法螺妙音吉祥，故八宝又称八吉祥。图中八宝众星捧寿，寓意："八宝呈吉祥，万寿自无疆。"

Since Buddhism was introduced to China in the Han Dynasty, Buddhist instruments became objects of good luck. The eight magic objects refer to the triton, the Wheel of the Law, the magic canopy, the magic shield, the lotus flower, the magic bottle, the gold fish, and the knitting knot. As the triton produces beautiful and auspicious sounds, the eight magic objects are also called the eight auspicious things. As the eight objects surround longevity, the message is that longevity is guaranteed because the eight magic objects bring good luck.

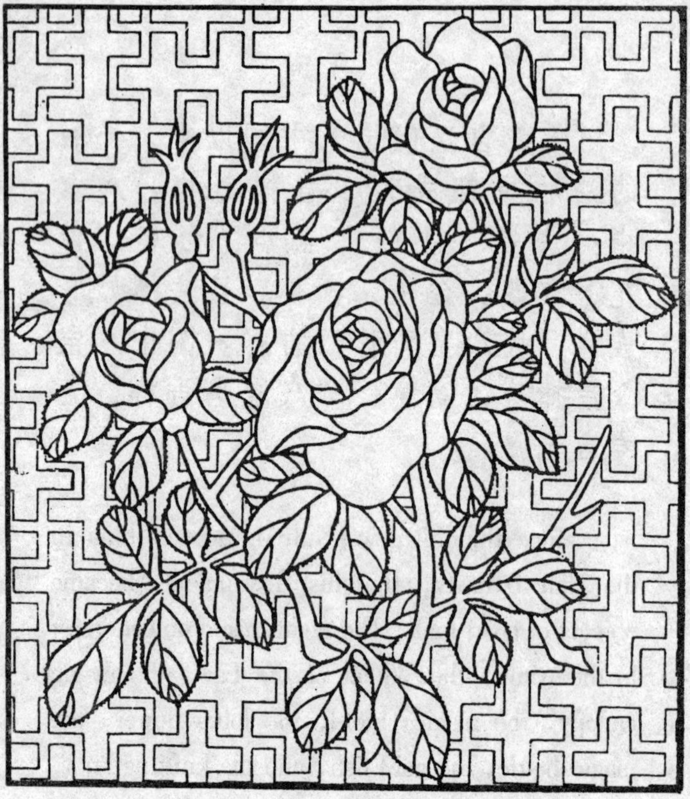

万代常春

10000 *generations of offsprings*

蔓，是带状植物茎，以“蔓带”谐音“万代”。或以“卐”字寓“万代”。月季花，又称长春花，四时艳丽，被誉为“花中皇后”，示“长春”。“万代长春”成一葫芦状，葫芦谐音为“福禄”、“护禄”。《伏羲考》：“汉族以葫芦为伏羲女娲本身。”多子也。

The vines in the picture form a pun with “10,0 00 generations”. The symbol 卐 may also appear in such pictures for its association with 10,000 generations. Chinese roses, bright in colors and blooming all year round, are hailed “queen of flowers”. The four Chinese characters for 10, 000 generations of offsprings are in the shape of a bottle gourd which is another pun with good fortune and salary. Bottle gourds have numerous seeds (association with children) and are regarded as the original combined body of the Chinese ancestors.

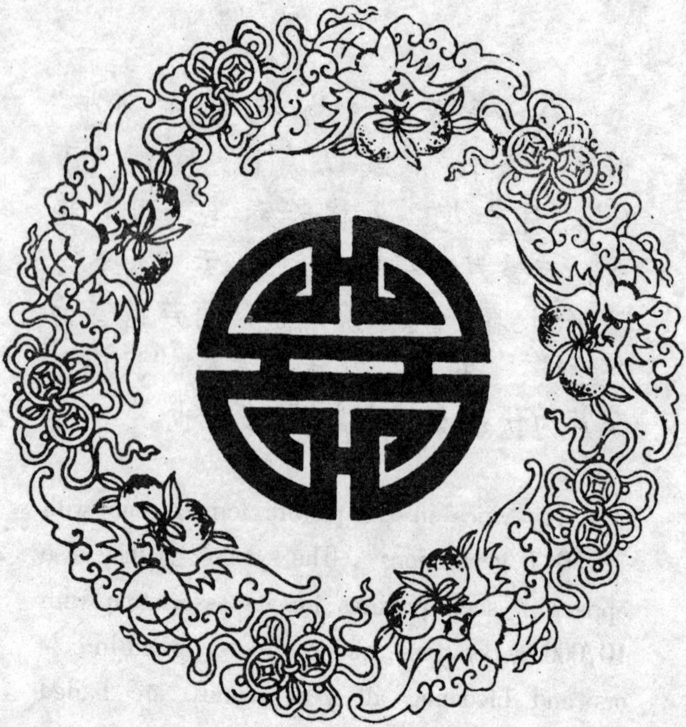

万寿无疆

A long lasting life

《诗经》中有六处出现万寿无疆。《诗·豳风·七月》："跻彼公堂，称彼兕斛，万寿无疆！"这里的万寿无疆，是指颂祝丰年无穷。后来用为祝寿之词。北宋·欧阳修《圣节五方老人祝寿文》："亿万斯年，共祝无疆之寿。"

The phrase "a long lasting life" appeared six times in the *Book of Songs*. Yet the meaning then and there is a wish for a good harvest. The phrase evolved to be an eulogy for longevity and was used in literature by many famous writers and poets. Literally, it means to live for 10,000 years.

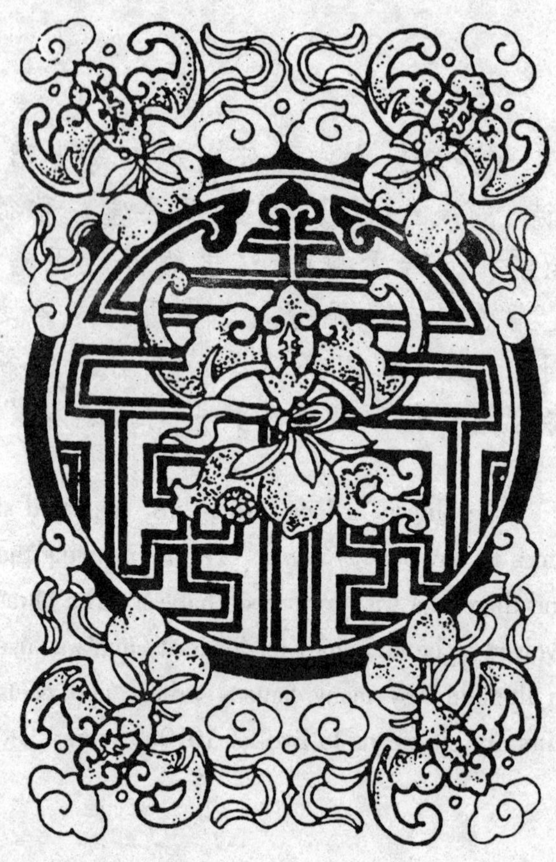

万寿五福

Longevity and five blessings

图案由五福捧寿、福寿三多、万寿团字几种吉祥纹样组成，寓意万年长寿、五福安康。中间的大团万寿字，表示五福捧寿寿为中心，福寿三多以寿为首。古人认为“人在一切在”，与基督教、佛教不同，中国人更看重今生今世。

The design is a combination of several good luck patterns all featuring good fortune, longevity, and salary. The implication is longevity to 10,000 years and peace, health, and blessings. The large character "longevity" in the center explains that a long life is of greater significance than any other blessings. Ancient Chinese believed humans were the basis of everything and the present life was their focus. Chinese seem not to share the Christian or Buddhist notions of an afterlife.

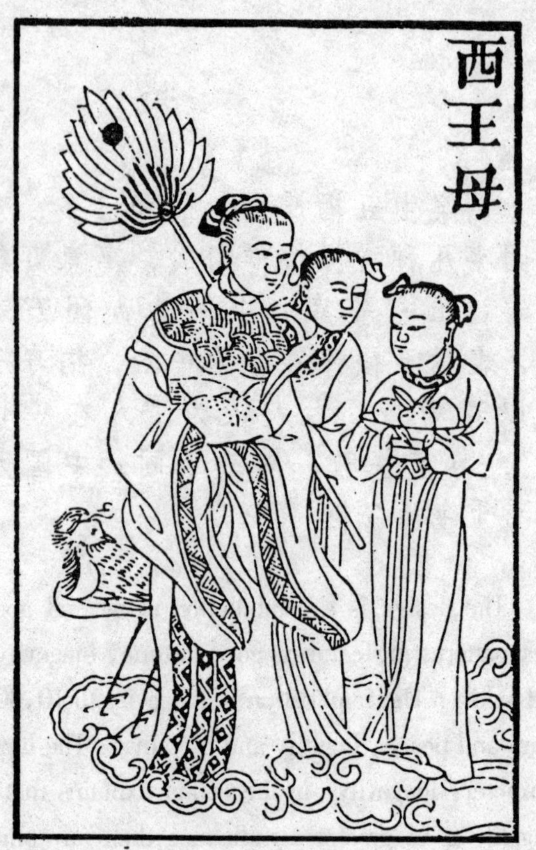

王母祝寿

Birthday celebrations for Hsi Wang Mu

传说每逢旧历三月初三，王母娘娘过生日之时，便在天宫瑶池举行蟠桃盛会，各路尊神、各界大仙应邀前往，品桃祝寿，是仙界的一大盛事。蟠桃三千年生实，品可长生不老。王母娘娘又名是西王母，是天界第一夫人。

It is said that March 3rd (lunar calendar) is the birthday of Hsi Wang Mu, the Queen Mother of the West. The Queen Mother would then hold a grand flat peach party at her heavenly palace where gods and immortals from all schools would come at her invitation to taste the peaches and congratulate her. It takes 3,000 years for the flat peach trees to bear fruits and the fruits have the power of turning one immortal. Hsi Wang Mu is the First Lady in heaven.

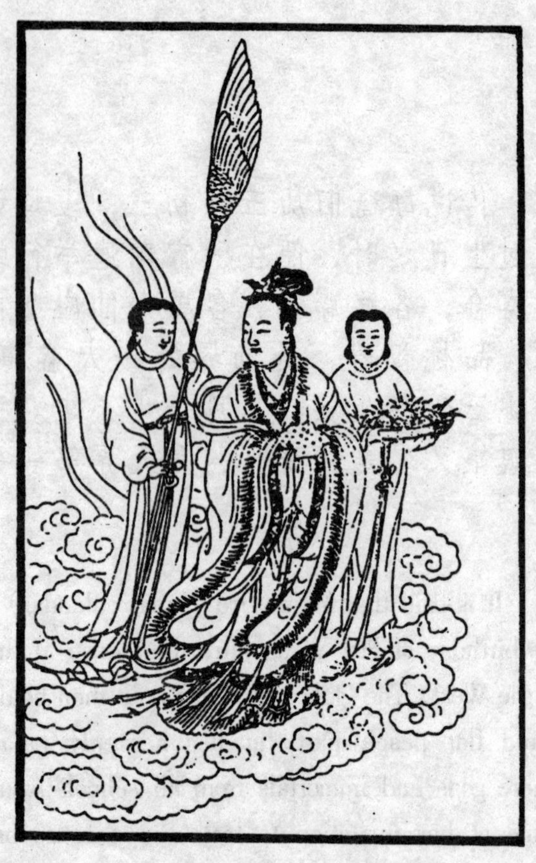

王母赐寿

Longevity bestowed by Hsi Wang Mu

王母娘娘是长寿仙人，被道家尊为女仙之宗。在汉代，民间就把她看成是赐福、赐寿、赐子、化灾的仙人。汉·焦延寿《易林》：“稷为尧使，西见王母。拜请百福，赐我善子。引船牵头，虽拘无忧。王母善祷，祸不成灾。”

Hsi Wang Mu is an immortal of eternal life and respected as the ancestor of fairies in Taoism. In the Han Dynasty, she was regarded by the common folks as the fairy that grants good fortune, longevity, children, and eliminates disasters. Her many capabilities are best illustrated in the work of Jiao Yanshou from the Han Dynasty.

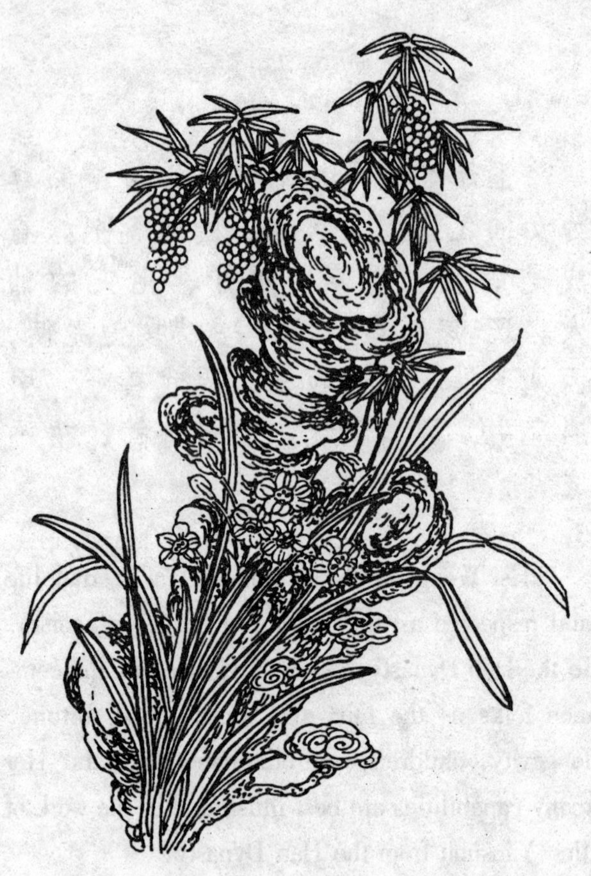

天仙寿芝

Fairies and longevity

太湖石、灵璧石、英石、黄蜡石是中国园林的四大名石。《博物志》："地以石为界。"石是永恒的，故有寿石之称。天竹取其"天"，水仙取其"仙"，合为"天仙"。灵芝仙草，食之可长寿。又"竹"谐音"祝"，亦有"天仙祝寿"之意。

Of the many stones extensively used in Chinese gardens, four types are most famous. Stones last and for this reason, are called longevity stones. Daffodils carry the "immortal" sound in Chinese. The glossy ganoderma are fairy plants that give people long life. "Bamboo" and "congratulation" sound the same in Chinese. The stones and different plants in the picture combine to form an eulogy for long life.

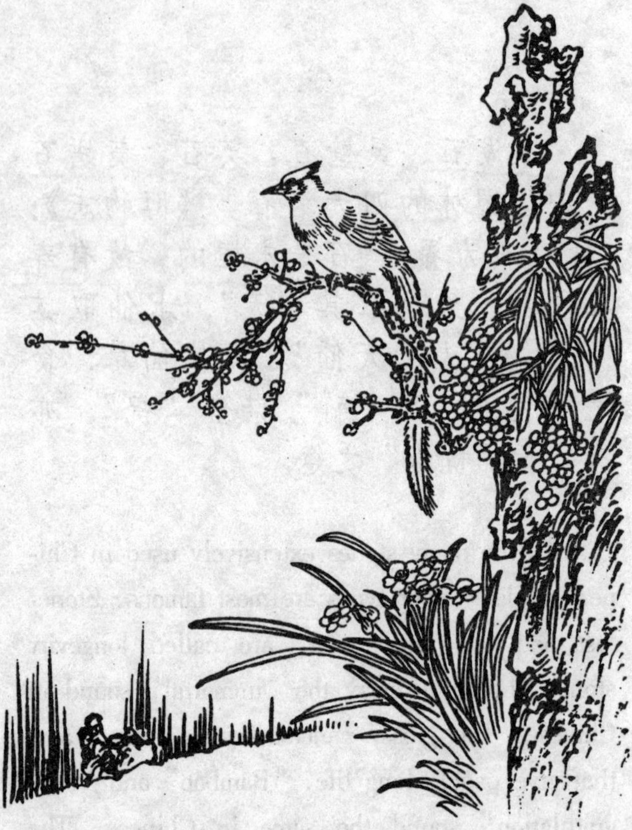

天仙拱寿

Fairies and longevity

天竹的“天”与水仙的“仙”，合为“天仙”。梅有“四德”，梅花五瓣，以示“五福”。梅拱托着绶鸟，“绶”与“寿”谐音，合为“拱寿”。另石亦为寿石。绶鸟在吉祥图中是长寿的瑞禽。又绶带是官吏身份、品级的标志，故也是禄位、富贵的象征。

Several plants are seen in this picture: nandina and daffodils, which together stand for fairies, a plum flower that has four virtues and its five petals coincide with the five blessings. There is also the long-tailed flycatcher, whose Chinese name includes the sound "longevity". And the stones are longevity stones. Long-tailed flycatcher typically appears in good luck pictures as an auspicious bird for longevity. A ribbon (a pun in Chinese with longevity) is also the symbol of official status and rank. So the second implication of this picture is salary and rank.

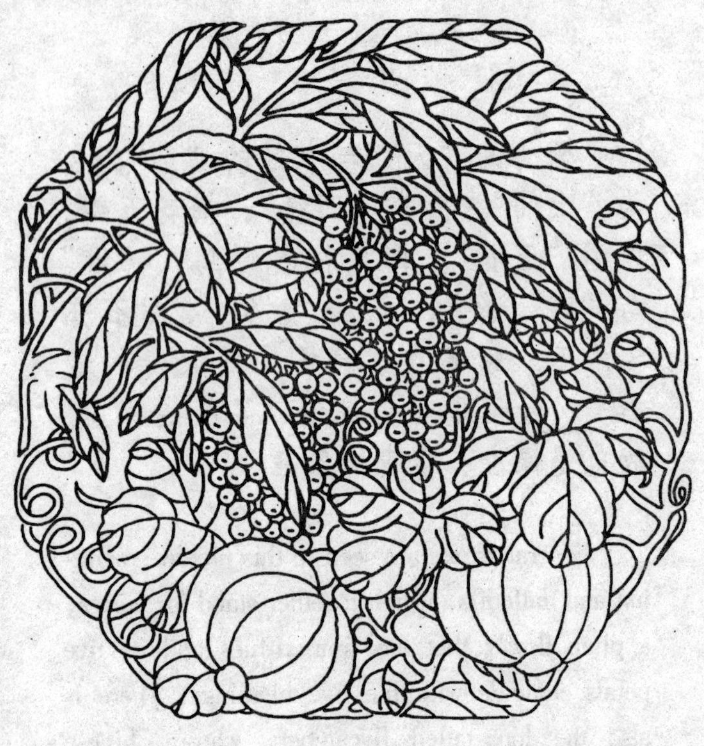

天地长久

Enduring as heaven and earth

《诗·大雅·绵》：“绵绵瓜瓞，民之初生，自土沮漆。”意为周朝的祖先像瓜瓞一样，世世相传，代代相继。图中天竹取其“天”，瓜瓞卧地而生取其“地”，瓜蔓绵长取其长久，合为“天地长久”。寓意家业兴旺，或夫妻天长地久。

Ancient Chinese literature compares the ancestors and offsprings of the Zhou Dynasty to continuous melon vines that pass from generation to generation with no stop. Nandina in the picture has the character “heaven” in it and melon vines grow on the ground “earth”. The message is a wish for family prosperity or lasting devotion between spouses.

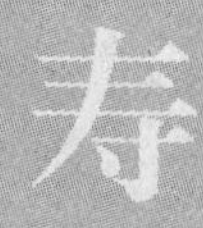

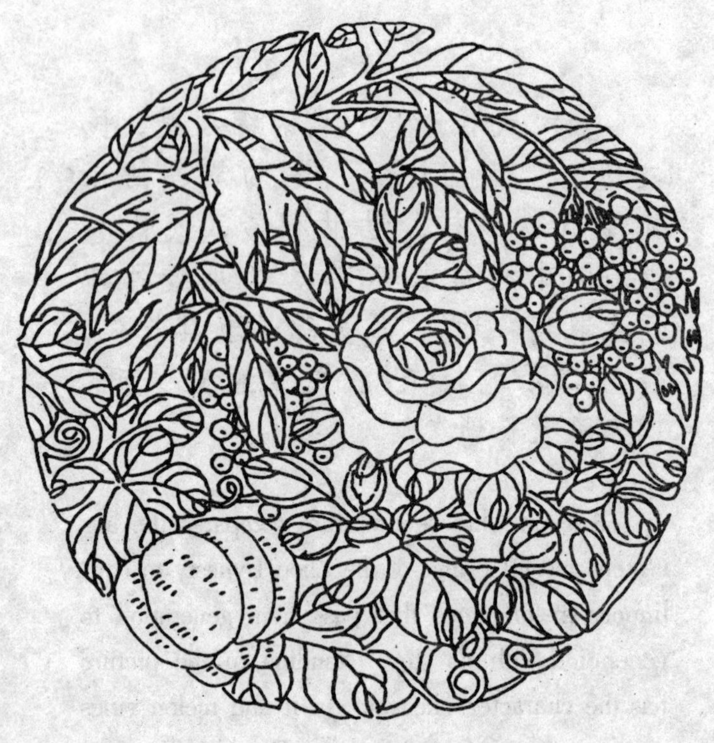

天地长春

Lasting as heaven and earth

《管子·白心》：“苞物众者，莫大于天地。”《镜花缘》：“四时有不谢之花，八节有长青之草。”图中的天竹、地瓜自示“天地”，月季花又称长春花，取其“长春”，合为“天地长春”。上有天下有地，人居其中，愿人与天地一样长春永在。

There is nothing more accommodating than heaven and earth. Here in the picture, nandina and sweet potatoes represent heaven and earth, and Chinese roses stand for lasting as they bloom all year round. Together with many flowers and plants that last a long time, man lives on the earth under heaven. May all men have lasting youth and endure forever like heaven and the earth.

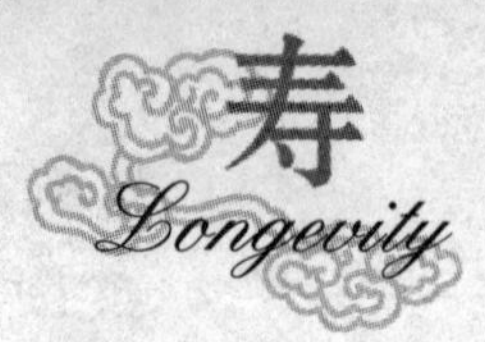

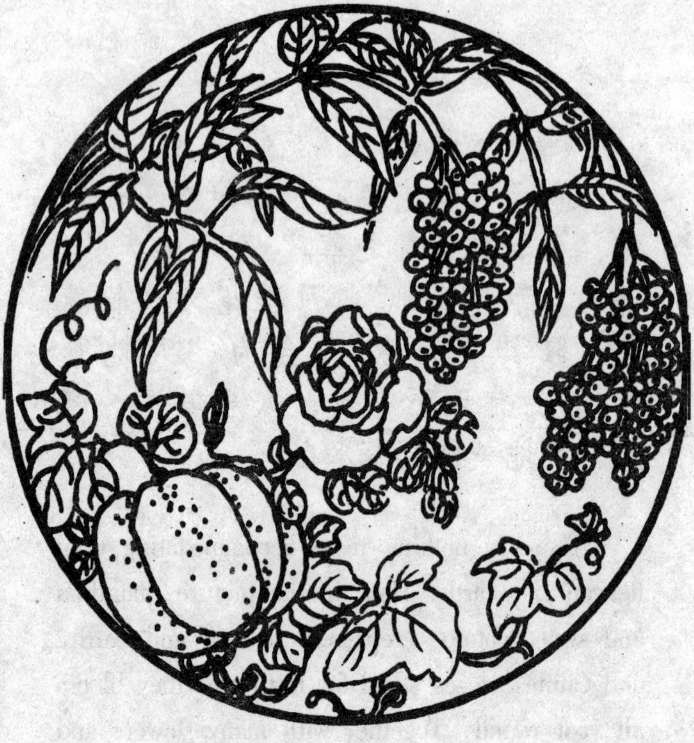

天地长春

Lasting as heaven and earth

图中以天竹示“天”，以地瓜示“地”，而月季花又名长春花，示“长春”。《群芳谱》：月季，“一名长春花”。《易经》：“天地氤氲，万物化醇。”苏辙《转对状》：“天之所生，地之所产，足以养人。”只有天地长春，人才能长久幸福。

Here in the picture, nandina and sweet potatoes represent heaven and earth, and Chinese roses stand for permanency as they bloom all year round. As literature from the Zhou and Song dynasties pictures for us, heaven and earth provide all the things man needs to live and multiply. An ever youthful heaven and earth are the basis for the lasting happiness of man.

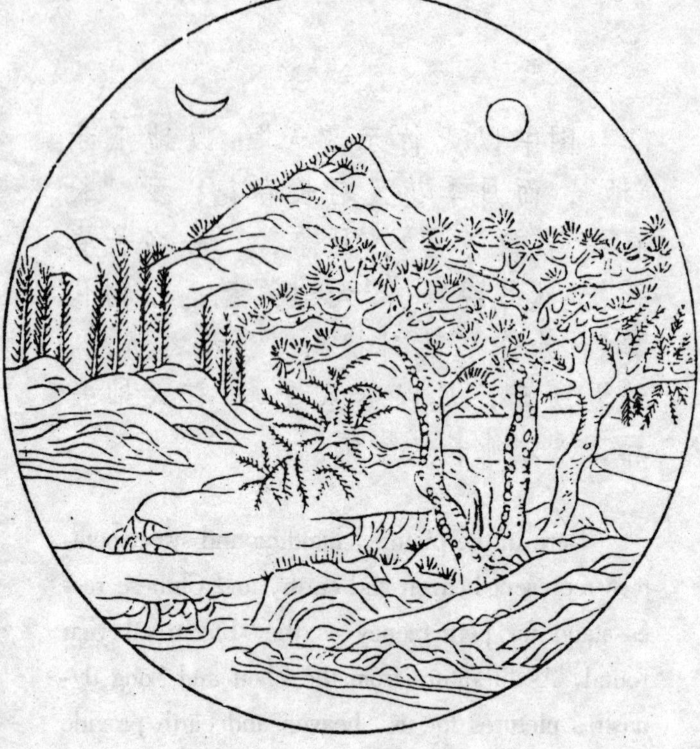

天保九如

An eulogy of nine comparisons

天保，是《诗·小雅》的篇名。《诗序》："下报上也。"是一首为君主祝福的诗。九如：如山、如阜、如陵、如岗、如川之方至、如月之恒、如日之升、如松柏之茂、如南山之寿。每句有如，故称"九如"，天保九如多做颂词。

Tianbao is the title of a piece of ancient literature that sings benediction to the Kings and Lords. The nine longevity comparisons are: like mountains and mounds, like mounts and uninterrupted stretches of hills, like rivers flowing over from afar, like the eternity of the moon, like the rise of the sun, like the longevity of Mount Zhongnanshan, like the exuberant pines and cypresses. The phrase is usually an eulogy.

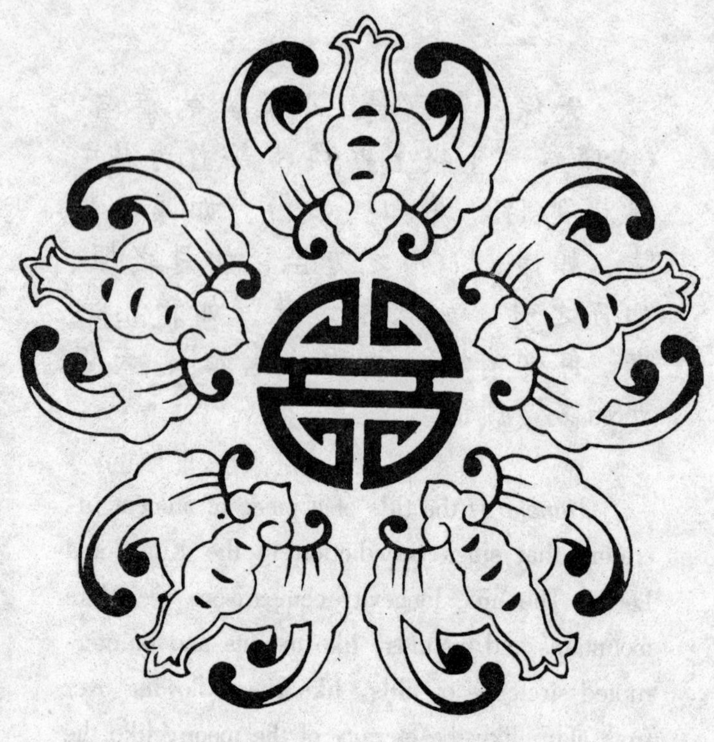

五福捧寿

Longevity held up by the five blessings

福、禄、寿、喜、财，是民间所称的五福，寿为五福之首。图中五只蝙蝠寓意五福，紧紧围绕着一个大团寿字，形成五福捧寿。《列子·天瑞》："天生万物，唯人为贵。"古人认为人在天地中，人在一切在，故五福唯寿为重。

Headed by longevity, the five blessings cherished by the common folks are good fortune, salary and position, longevity, happiness, and wealth. Five bats in the picture imply the five blessings. A large rounded Chinese character "longevity" and five bats closely surrounding it form the picture of longevity held up by the five blessings. As ancient people regarded man as the most essential part of nature, top priority was directed to longevity.

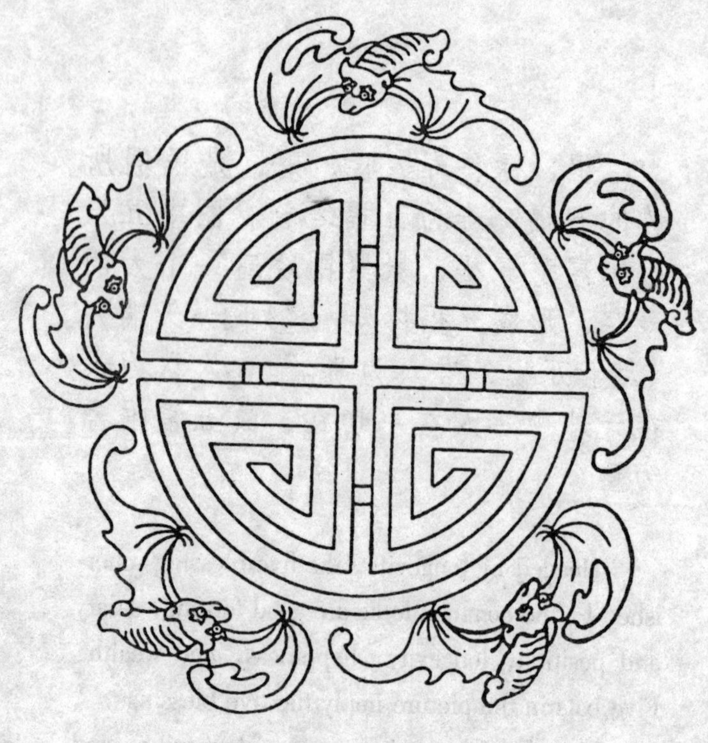

五福捧寿

Longevity held up by the five blessings

《抱朴子》："千岁蝙蝠，色如白雪，集则倒悬，脑重故也。此物得而阴干服之，令人寿万岁。"蝙蝠为长寿之禽。民间传说蝙蝠为老鼠吃盐所变，故又称"飞鼠"、"仙鼠"。因"蝠"与"福"谐音，在吉祥图中蝙蝠多表示"福"。

Ancient Chinese records tell people that there is a kind of white bat that has grown for 1,000 years. It hangs upside down to rest due to the overwhelming weight of its brains. Those who get to eat it can live up to 10,000 years. Bats are animals with a long life. Folk stories go that bats are transformed from rats that have eaten salt, which is why bats also go as flying rats, and fairy rats. In good luck pictures, bats represent "blessing" as a pun in Chinese.

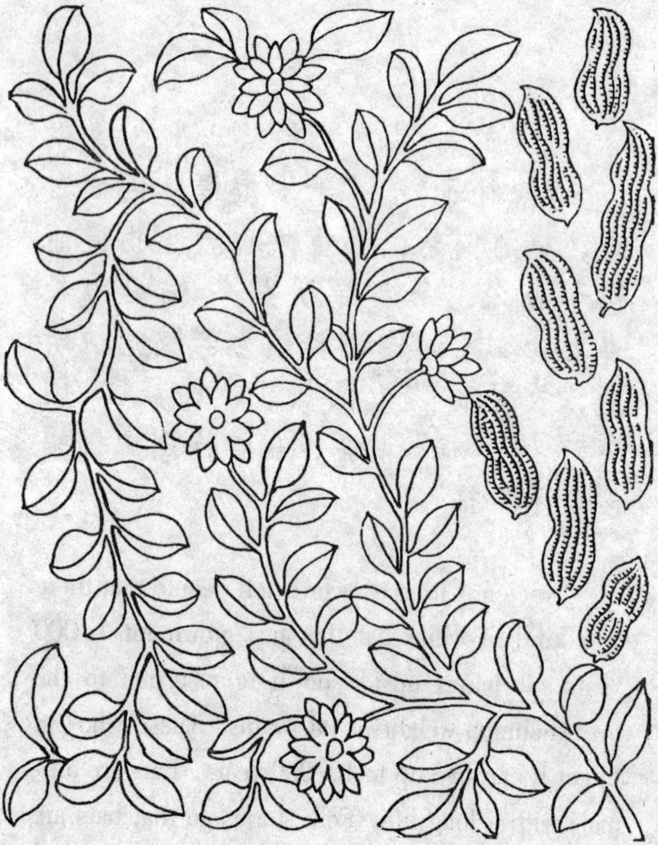

长生不老

Live forever

and never grow old

汉·无名氏《古诗十九首·驱车上东门》："人生忽如寄，寿无金石固。万岁更相送，圣贤莫能度。"曹操感："人生几何。"李白慨："朝如青丝暮如雪。"图中的落花生，简称花生，俗称长生果，果实房中有子。民间喻为子孙不断或长生不老。

An anonymous Han Dynasty poet laments over the limited length of life man can enjoy on the earth: "Life does not stay on forever as gold and stones do, and this is the same for all sages". Cao Cao of the Three Kingdoms Period and Li Bai of the Tang Dynasty shared the same view. Peanuts, also called longevity nuts, bear seeds (a pun with children) in their nuts. People associate peanuts with continuity of offsprings or longevity without getting old.

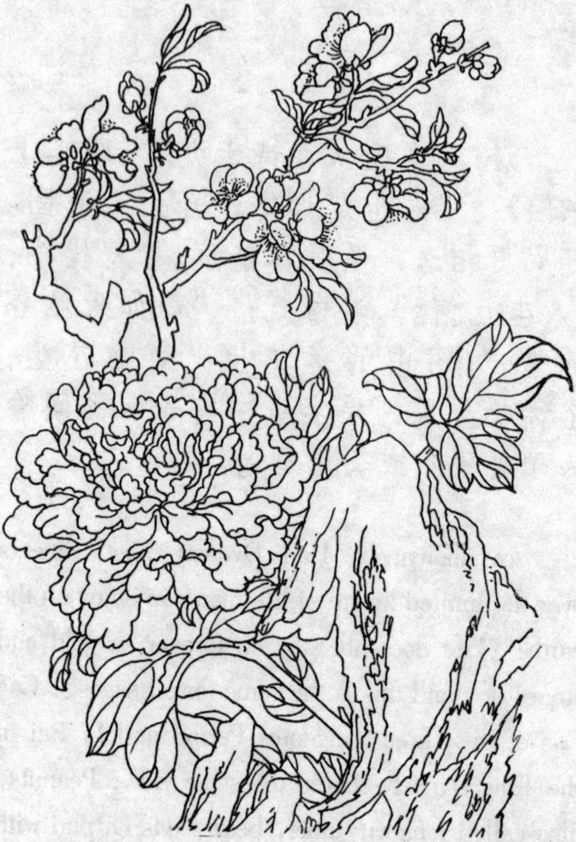

长命富贵

Longevity and wealth

唐·白行简《望夫石赋》："最坚者石，最灵者人；何精诚之所感，忽变化而如神。"石，又称寿石，在吉祥图中多喻长寿、长命等。古来诗人、画家、书法家多有好石者。图中牡丹花，又称富贵花，取其"富"。桂花谐音取其"贵"。

As a poet from the Tang Dynasty said: the sturdiest of all is the stone, and the most intelligent of all is man. Stones, also called longevity stones, appear in good luck pictures to imply longevity. Many ancient poets, painters, and calligraphists were fond of stones and stone collection. The peony flowers in the picture indicate wealth and sweet-scented osmanthus high official ranking.

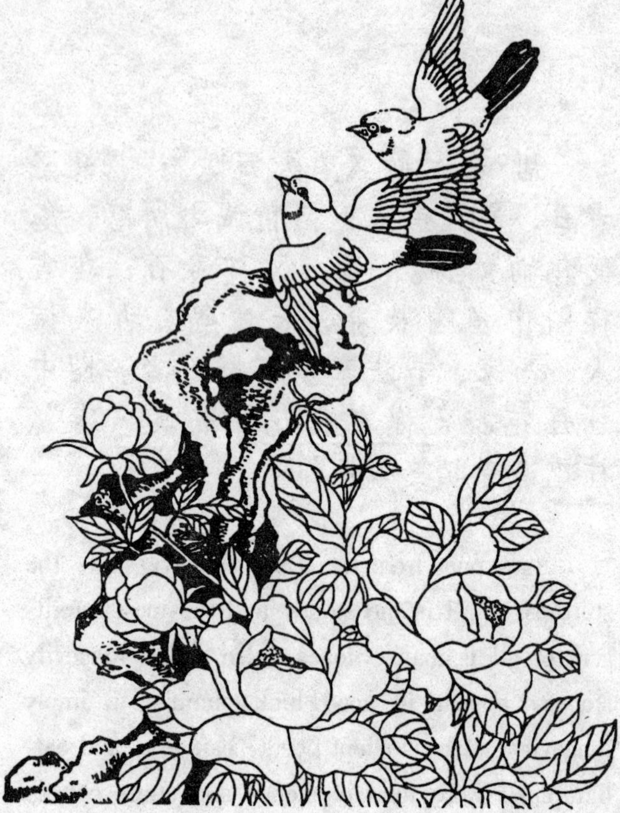

长春白头

Stay together till their hair turns white

长春白头，指夫妻偕老，青春永在。元·郑庭玉《古今杂剧·宋上皇御断金凤钗》：“动不动拍着手当街里叫，你想看几场儿，厮守的白头到老。”图中月季花，又名长春花，喻“长春”。白头翁鸟，老鸟头毛全变白，喻白头偕老。

The phrase for “stay together till white hair appears” appeared in a Chinese drama of the Yuan Dynasty. The Chinese roses in the picture stand for eternal spring. The hair in the head of Chinese bulbuls turns all white when they get old, hence the bird is used in association with devoted spouses whose hair has turned white after all the years.

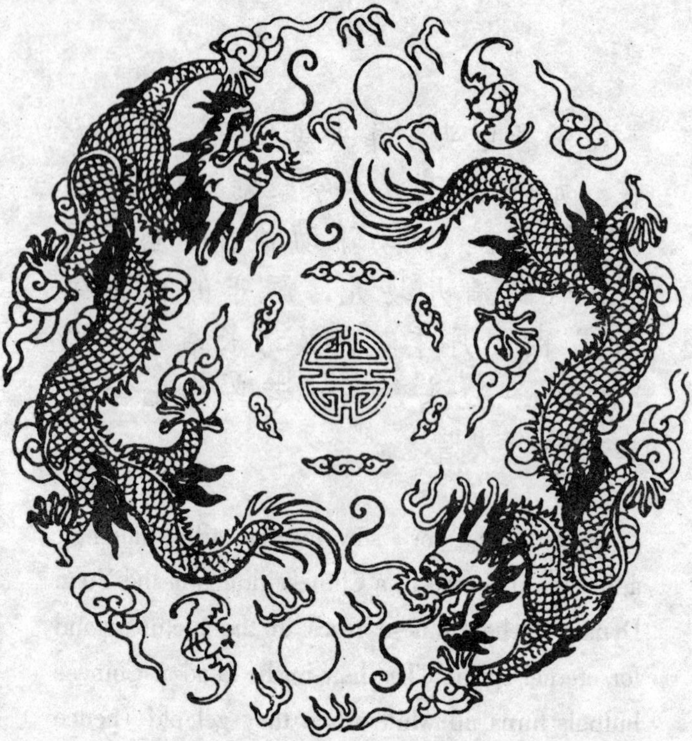

双龙拱寿

Longevity supported by two dragons

《说文解字》："龙，鳞虫之长，能幽能明，能细能巨，能短能长。春分而升天，秋分而潜渊。"龙是动物的始祖，龙是最大的神物，龙是最大的吉祥物，故帝王被称为"真龙天子。"龙的图案只为皇帝专用，现已走进寻常百姓家。

The *Origin of Chinese Characters* states that the dragon is the head of all scaled creatures. It can be visible or concealed, tiny or giant, and short or long. It ascends to heaven at the Spring Equinox and hides up in deep water at the Autumn Equinox. The dragon is the ancestor of animals, the largest divine animal, and the largest good luck creature, so the emperor is called the real dragon and the son of heaven. Exclusively reserved for emperors in the past, dragon designs have now become a common element in the life of ordinary people.

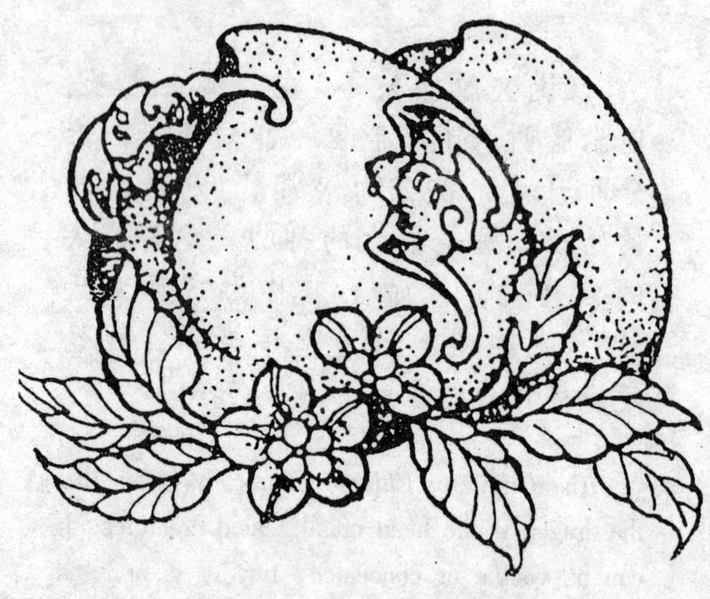

双福拱寿

Longevity supported by two blessings

《神农经》："玉桃服之长生不死。若不得早服之，临死服之，其尸毕天地不朽。"桃亦称寿桃，在吉祥图案中喻长寿。蝙蝠取其"福"音，在吉祥图案中喻福。福为吉祥之总，寿为最难得之福，"双福拱寿"寓意幸福、长寿成双。

A Chinese classical book on plants talks about a kind of magic peach: it turns living men into immortals and the bodies of the dying stay enduring if they eat the fruit. In good luck designs, peaches imply longevity. Bats share a pun with blessings and are symbols of such in good luck pictures. So two bats and a peach mean happiness and longevity in pairs.

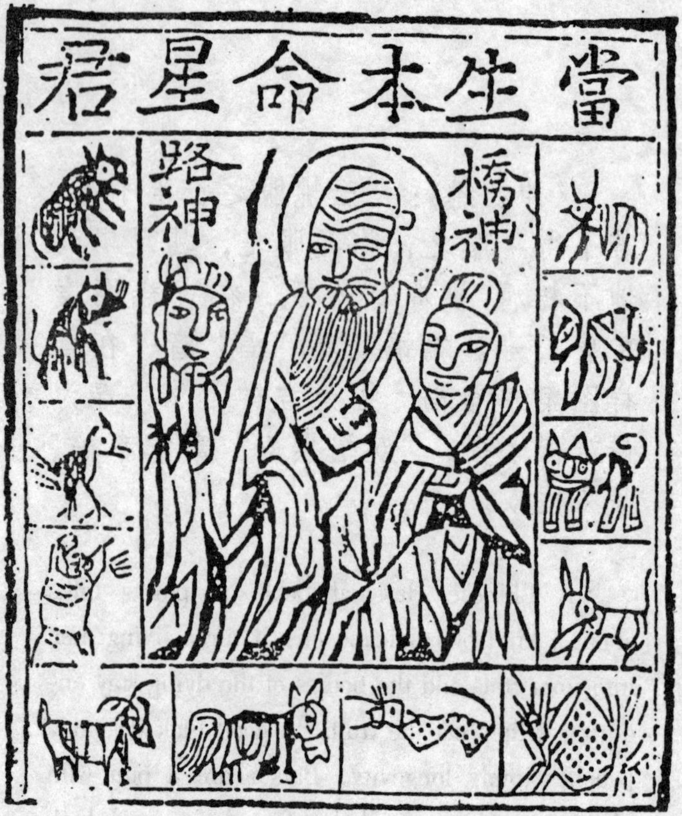

本命平安

Peace on one's birthday and in years represented by one's symbolic animal

中国人是很讲究“本命”的。“本命日”要过生日、祝寿。“本命年”要系红裤腰带，以驱凶避邪。本命年要拜乞本命星君，以顺利渡过“槛儿年”，求一生顺利，这叫“求顺星”。旧时记年用天干地支法，并有十二生肖相配。

Chinese make a point of observing longevity formalities on birthdays and in the years presided by the animals of the birth year. In the corresponding years, a red belt shall be worn on the waist to drive away the evil and evade the ominous. The stars over the years represented by different animals are to be worshipped for a smooth life. In the past, years were marked by the ten Heavenly Stems and the twelve Earthly Branches and matched by 12 animals.

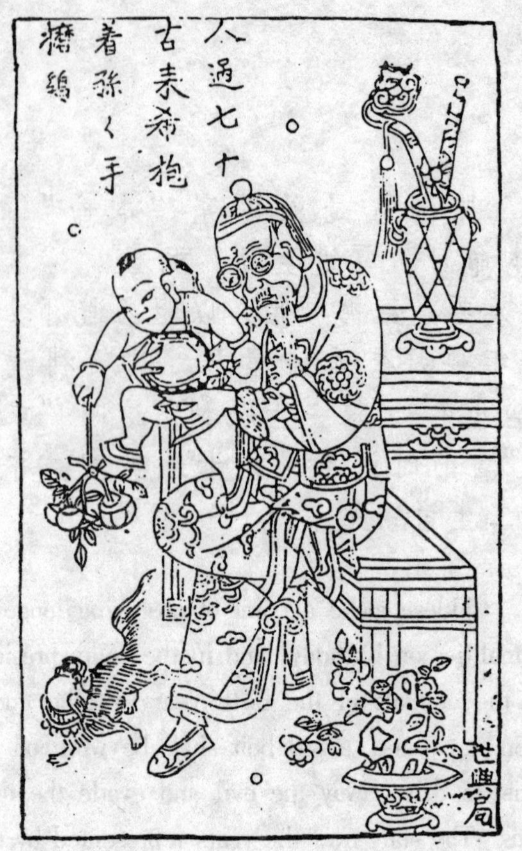

古稀之福

The good fortune of turning 70 years old

杜甫《曲江二首》："朝回日日典春衣，每日江头尽醉归；酒债寻常行处有，人生七十古来稀。穿花蛱蝶深深见，点水蜻蜓款款飞。传与风光共流转，暂时相赏莫相违。"人活七十，在古代甚为不易，含贻弄孙安享晚年。

A poem by Du Fu describes the beauty of summer time. In the poem is the famous sentence "the age of 70 has been a rarity since ancient times". At the age of 70, one can relax, chew on a piece of candy, play with one's little grandchildren, and enjoy what is remaining of one's life peacefully.

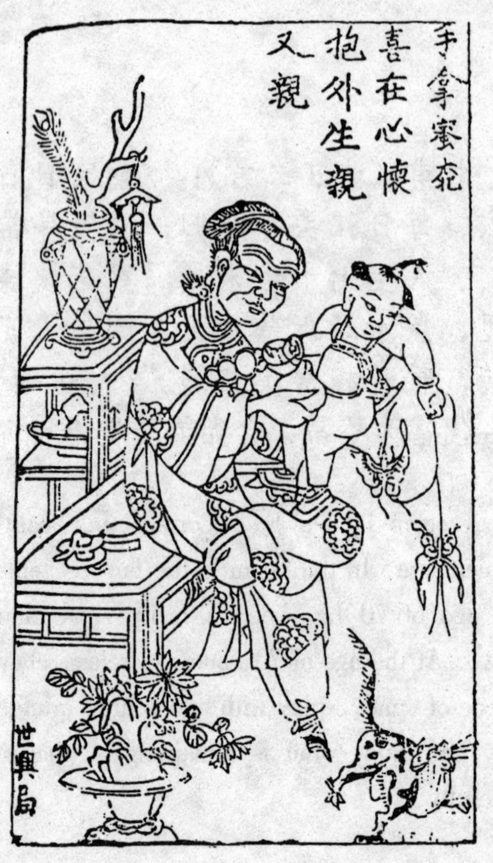

古稀之寿

A long life of 70 years

旧时有祝夫妇双寿联:“家中全福,天上双星。”“祝愿翁姥年年健,期望儿孙个个强。”“二老并高年不让神仙眷属,九畴衍洪范兼全福寿儿孙。”在古代,人活到七十稀有,是福、是寿。人奋斗了一生,到晚年要享天伦之乐。

In old times, some couplets were eulogies for the longevity of spouses. For example, “May the family be bestowed with all five blessings and may the husband and wife be both protected by the longevity star”, and “May the parents stay healthy while growing to an old age and may the children and grandchildren grow up strong”, etc. In ancient times, not many people lived to 70 years of age. Because of this, it was regarded as an age of longevity and good fortune. Surely one deserves some good rest after a full life's hard work and struggle.

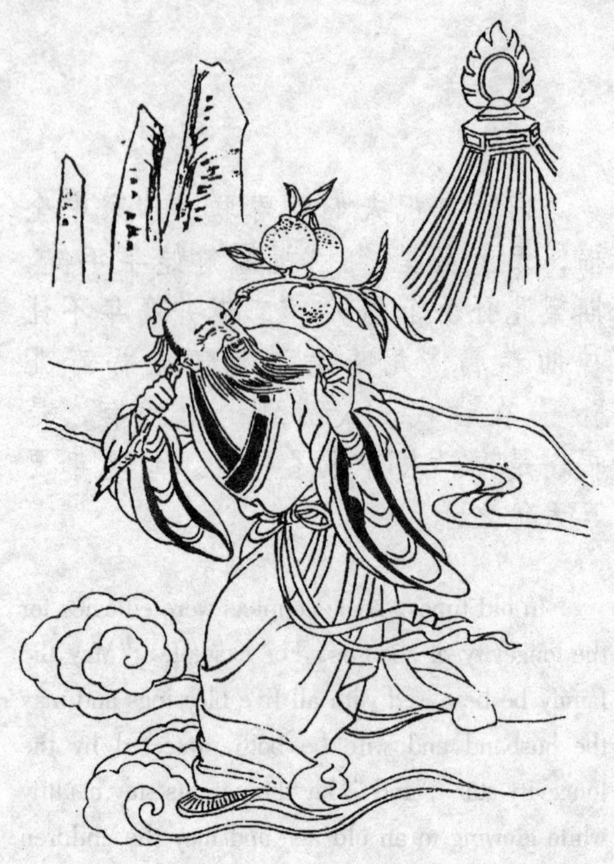

东方朔捧桃

Dongfang Shuo presents flat peaches

东方朔捧桃图，旧时多作祝寿之用。《刘仙传》："东方朔者，平原厌次人也，久在吴中，为书师数十年。武帝时上书说便宜，拜为郎……作深浅显然之行，或忠言或戏语，莫知其旨。"桃为西王母蟠桃，吃之可长生不老。

The picture featuring Dongfang Shuo presenting flat peaches is for birthday congratulations. Dongfang Shuo, a famous ancient scholar and court official, is known in history as a man of good humor. He was good at providing advice and reprimand to the emperor through funny stories or other forms that did not offend the royal majesty directly. The flat peaches shown in the picture are those grown on the trees of the Queen Mother of the West, which have the magic power of giving people eternal life.

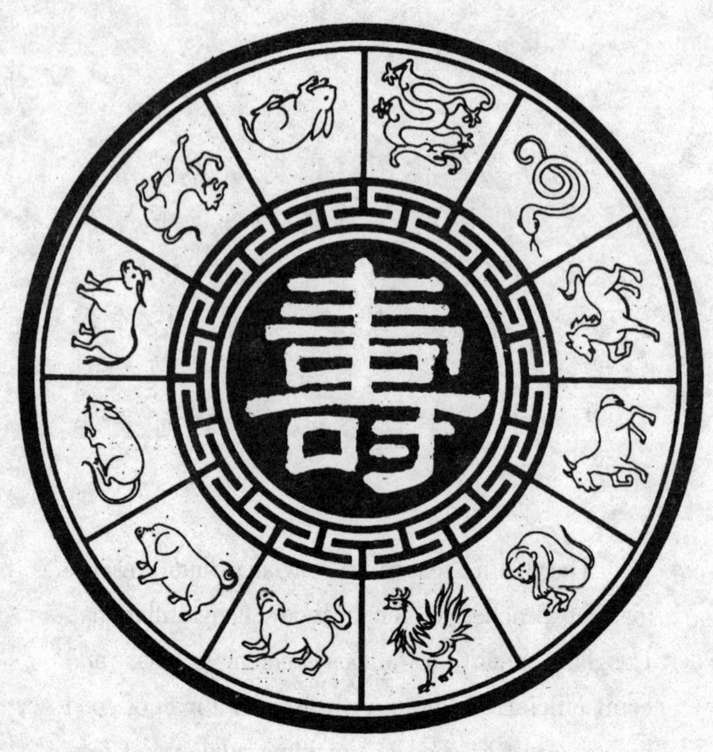

生肖贺寿

Birthday celebrations and the 12 symbolic animals

《诗经·小雅》："如南山之寿，不骞不崩。"寿为长久。《楚辞·天问》："延年不死，寿何所止?"寿为年长。《史记·高帝纪》："高祖奉玉卮，起为太上皇寿。"寿为祝人长寿。"生肖庆寿"是天增岁月人增寿之意。

The notion of longevity has been talked about and aspired to by the Chinese since very ancient times. As time advances and a year is added each year, man gets older and this is something worth congratulating. As each of the 12 animals represents a year, having them in pictures of birthday congratulations is in line with the theme.

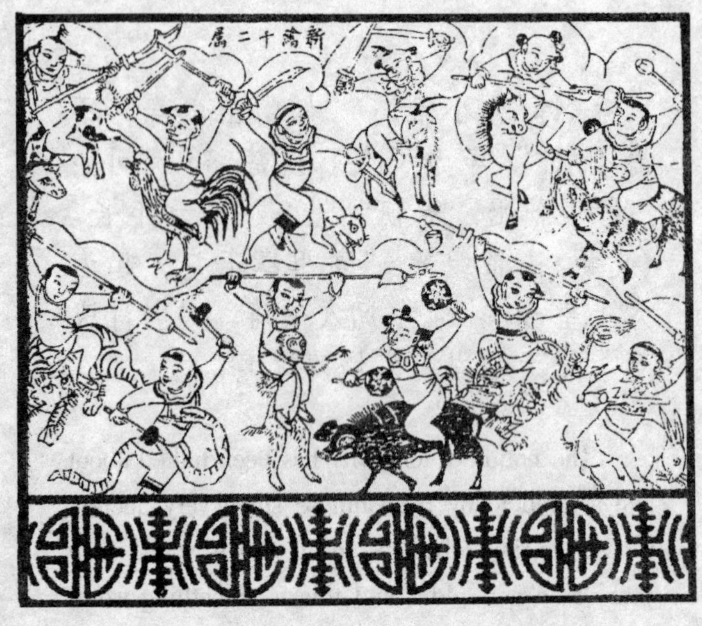

生肖贺寿

Birthday celebrations and the 12 symbolic animals

子鼠、丑牛、寅虎、卯兔、辰龙、巳蛇、午马、未羊、申猴、酉鸡、戌狗、亥猪。十二生肖即以十二地支配十二种动物。十二生肖在古代又称十二禽、十二兽、十二属、十二神等。寿为五福之首，生肖贺寿、本命平安为大吉。

Ancient Chinese astrologists matched the 12 Earthly Branches (signs of order) with 12 animals: the first is the rat, the second the ox, the third the tiger, the fourth the hare, the fifth the dragon, the sixth the snake, the seventh the horse, the eighth the sheep, the nineth the monkey, the 10th the rooster, the 11th the dog, and the 12th the boar. In ancient times, the 12 animals were called the 12 birds, the 12 beasts, and the 12 gods, etc. As longevity is the top of the five blessings, great fortunate events in life surely include a peaceful life and many birthday celebrations.

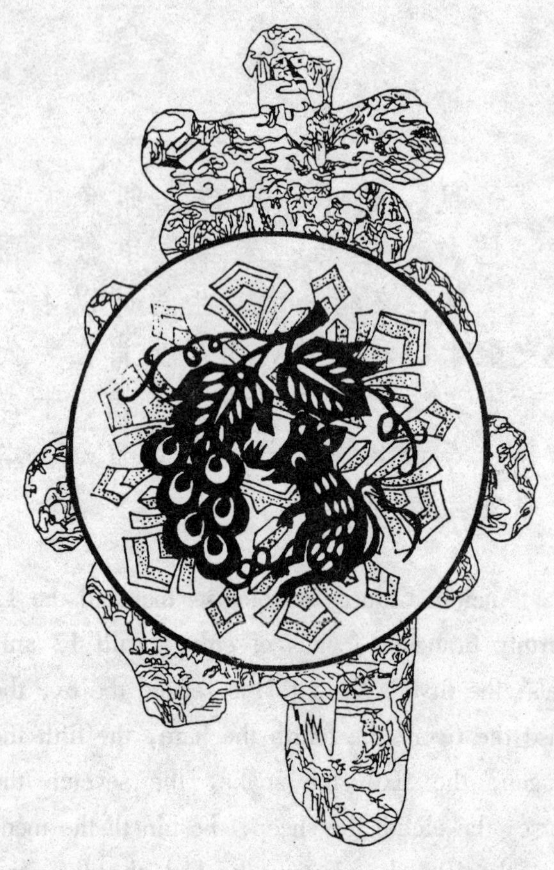

子鼠贺寿

The rat congratulates one's birthday

天年鼠年首，天月鼠月首，天时鼠时首。相传轩辕黄帝遴选十二生肖，报名参赛的动物颇多。比赛中众兽奔腾、一牛当先，快到终点时，偷骑在牛背上的鼠却一跃居前，成为生肖之首。人生五福当推寿，子鼠居首合献诗。

The rat is the first of all the years in the 12 Earthly Branches. It is said that lots of animals responded to the invitation of the Yellow Emperor, the first legendary emperor in China, to be chosen as the 12 representative animals. As the beasts raced to arrive for registration, the ox took the lead. But just before the ox made it, the rat, who had been hiding on the ox's back, jumped forward to become No. One. As longevity leads the rest of the five blessings, the No. One rat presents a poem of congratulations.

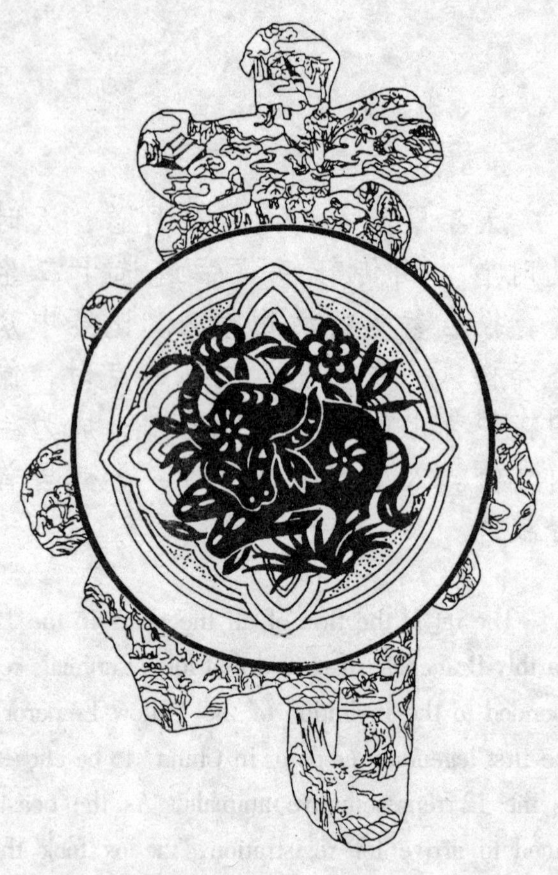

丑牛贺寿

The ox congratulates one's birthday

《清异录》："有田老不喜杀牛，曰：'天下人吃用，皆从此黄毛菩萨身上发生'"。"黄毛菩萨"则成了牛的雅号。《七修类稿》："凡草不经牛啖之必茂。"在陕西一些地方的民俗，将为老年人庆生、祝寿称为"赶牛王会"。

Historical records tell us that there was an elder by the name Tian who hated killing oxen for this reason: all that supports mankind comes from the body of this yellow-haired Buddha. Yellow-haired Buddha thus became the name of oxen. In some areas in Shaanxi Province, the local people refer to birthday celebrations for elders as "go to the fair of the ox king".

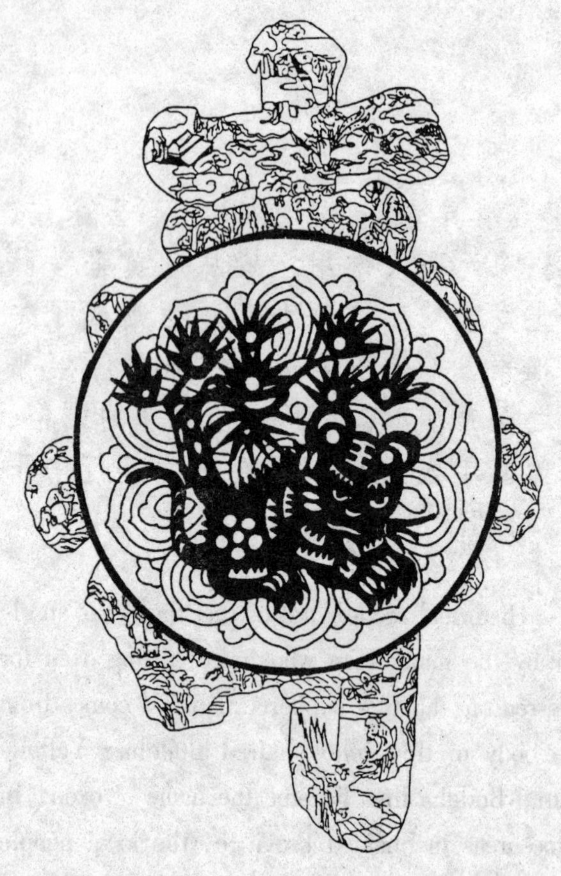

寅虎贺寿

The tiger congratulates one's birthday

《春秋运斗枢》："枢星散而为虎。"《宋书》："白虎，王者不暴虐，则白虎仁，不害物。"《抱朴子》："虎及鹿兔皆寿千岁，满五百岁者其色皆白。"《风俗通》："虎者阳物，百兽之长也。"旧有寿联："虎威八面，桃寿三千。"贺寿语也。

Ancient Chinese historical books from the Song and other dynasties have the following account about tigers: tigers are transformed from the hub stars, that they are tamed and would not hurt anyone if the ruling emperor is not violent, and that together with the deer and hare, tigers can live to 1,000 years and their hair turns white at 500 years. It is also recorded that the tiger is the head of all the beasts. An old couplet says this: longevity to man and power to the tiger.

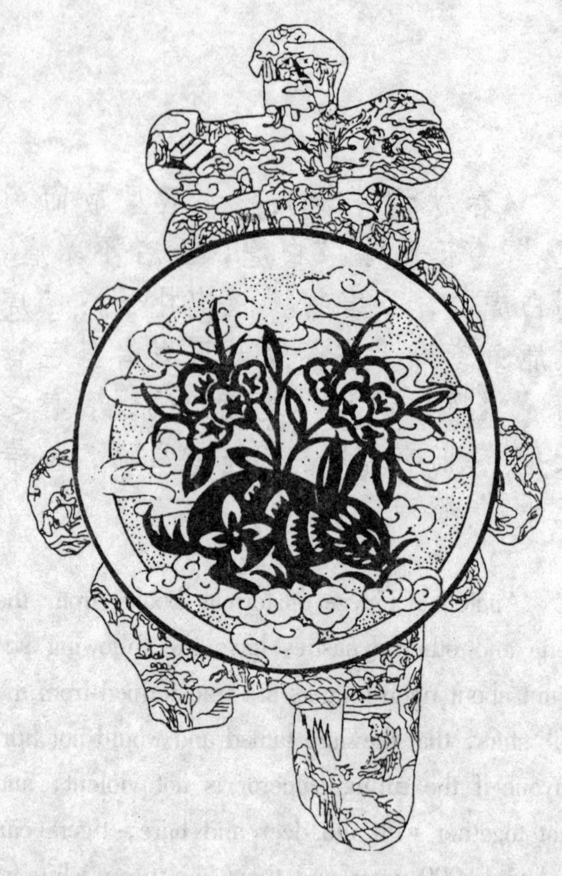

卯兔贺寿

The hare congratulates one's birthday

《抱朴子》：“兔寿千岁，五百岁其色白。”《陔余丛考》：“董昌以谶有‘兔子上金床’之语，谓己太岁在卯，遂以卯年卯月卯日即位。此见于五代时者也。”此为属兔者称帝之意。兔居月中乃神兽，卯兔贺寿，自是天赐遐龄。

Ancient Chinese literature tells us that the hare can live to 1,000 years and its hair turns white at 500 years. It also gives an account on how Dong Chang used a prophecy about the hare to win himself the position of emperor. The hare resides in the moon and is hence a divine beast. When the hare congratulates one's birthday, surely this is longevity bestowed by heaven.

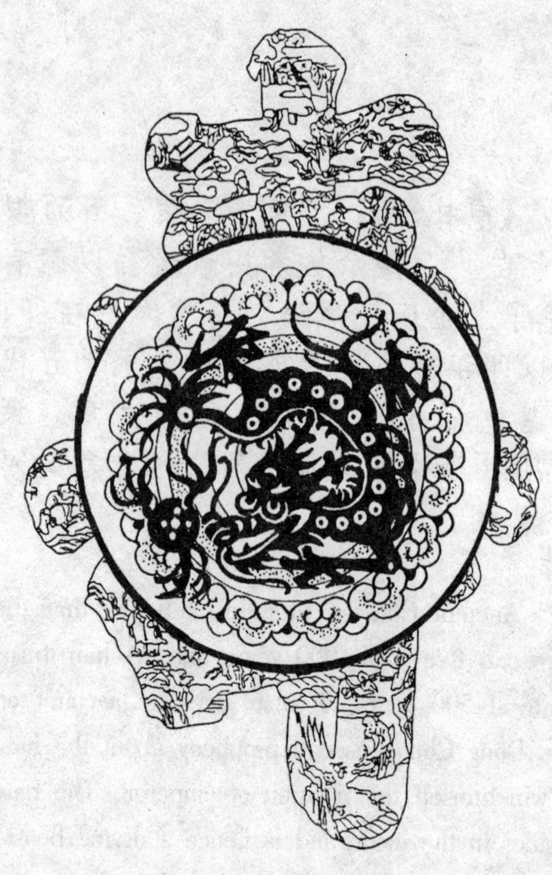

辰龙贺寿

The dragon congratulates one's birthday

飞龙在天，犹圣人之在王位。《说文》："龙，鳞虫之长，能幽能明，能细能巨，能短能长。春分而升天，秋分而潜渊。"《宋书》："赤龙，河图者，地之符也。王者德至渊泉，则河出龙图。"龙是万灵之长，是最大的吉祥物。

As dragons fly in the sky, wise men preside over states as kings. The *Origin of the Chinese Characters* states that dragon is the head of all scaled creatures. It can be visible or concealed, tiny or giant, and short or long. It ascends to heaven at the Spring Equinox and hides up in deep water at the Autumn Equinox. A book from the Song Dynasty says that red dragons, the signs of the earth, appear in rivers when the ruler is impressively virtuous. Dragon is the head of all creatures and the largest auspicious animal.

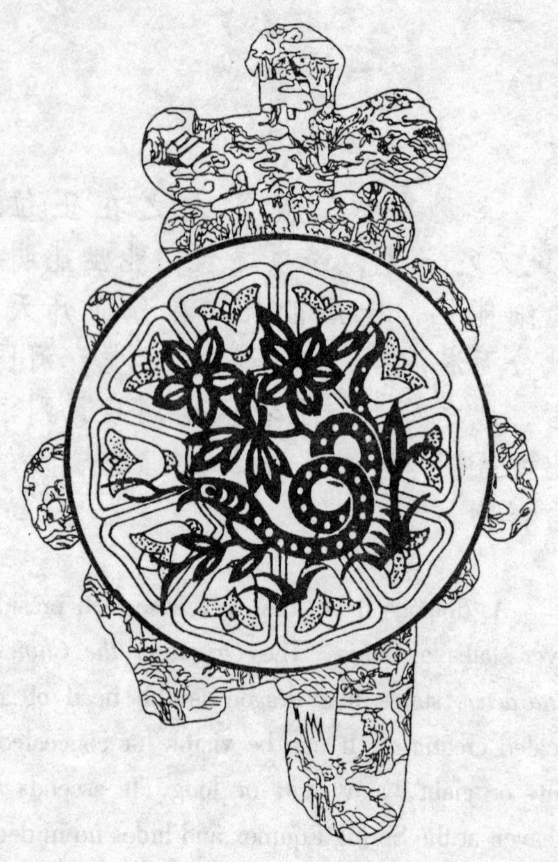

巳蛇贺寿

The snake congratulates one's birthday

《说文》："巳也，四月阳气已出，阴气已藏，万物见成文章，故巳为蛇象形。"蛇亦称小龙，有的地方把蛇奉为"青龙菩萨"，也有的地方把蛇称为"苍龙"或"家龙"。《水东日记》："俗择葬地以验蛇盘兔为上。"

The sixth in number, the snake represents April when nature is in basic harmony and shows itself in vivid forms. The snake is called the mini dragon and worshipped in some places as the green dragon Buddha. According to old customs, the best place for burying the dead is where snakes and hares live.

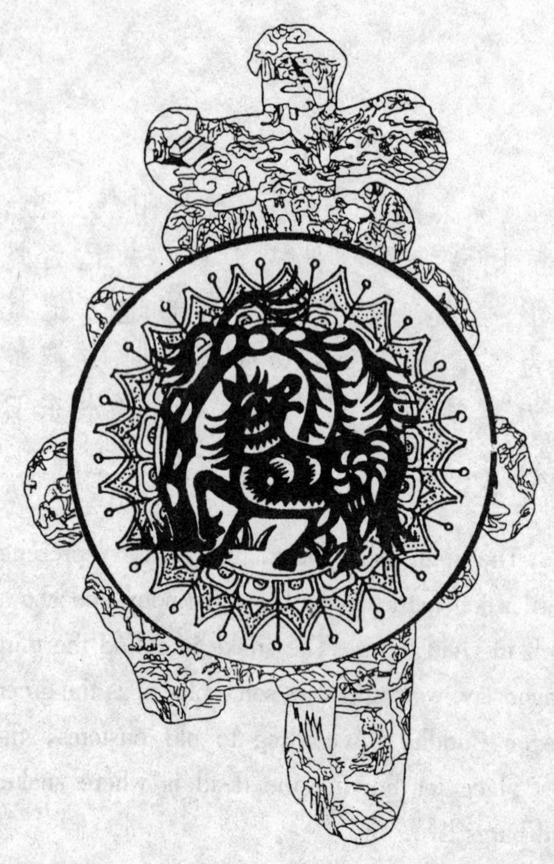

午马贺寿

The horse congratulates one's birthday

《抱朴子》："午日称三公者，马也。""午日三公"是古代文人送给马的雅号。李贺诗："此马非凡马，房星本是星。"古人以"房精"做为马的别名，并云"马为房星之精"。午为阳极之象，以马配午，阳气最盛。

The seventh in number, the horse is called the master of Wu by some ancient men of letters. Li He said in his poem: "This is no ordinary horse – it is the house star presiding over the property". This tells people ancient Chinese used to call horses "spirits of the house". Outward and strong are the traits of Wu and the horse is the best match for it.

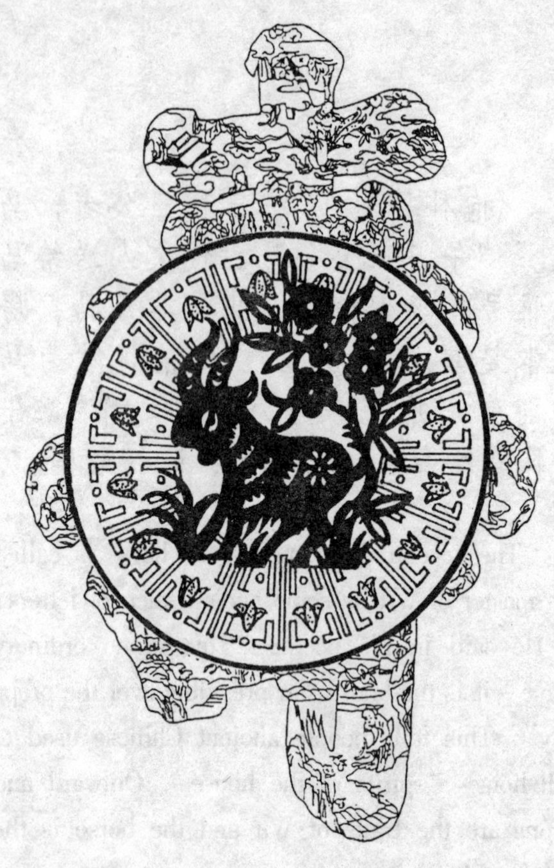

未羊贺寿

The sheep congratulates one's birthday

温顺、合群是羊的美德。华夏先民在上古过着游牧生活，羊肥美成群，是一件很“吉祥”的事，所以“吉祥”二字最早写成“吉羊”。《汉元嘉刀铭》：“宜侯王，大吉羊。”《玄中记》：“千岁之树精为青羊。”羊，长寿之征。

Obedience, mildness and gregariousness are the virtues of sheep. In ancient times, Chinese ancestors led a nomadic life and large groups of fat sheep were auspicious signs. For this reason, the earliest Chinese character for good luck had the image of a sheep in it. Some records state that spirits of trees that had lived for 1000 years became dark sheep. Sheep is the symbol of longevity.

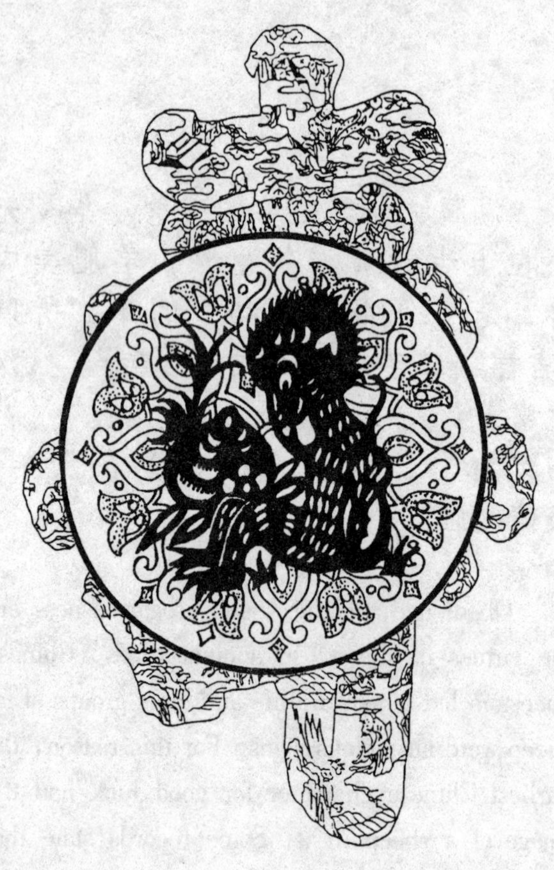

申猴贺寿

The monkey congratulates one's birthday

"猴桃瑞寿"图置于大寿字之中，大寿字中又有"八仙庆寿"、"群仙贺寿"等图，表示"申猴贺寿"。道教称铅为金母，并讲"真铅生庚"，天干庚辛为金，地支申酉也为金，猴是申的属相，猴也称之为"金公"，故多用"金猴"。

In the large longevity character in this picture is the design of "longevity, peaches, and the monkey" as well as other birthday congratulation pictures. In Taoism, both the seventh and eighth of the 10 Heavenly Stems and the ninth and 10th of the 12 Earthly Branches have traits of gold and the monkey, the ninth in order, is also called the "gold master". This is the reason why people tend to call the monkey the "gold monkey".

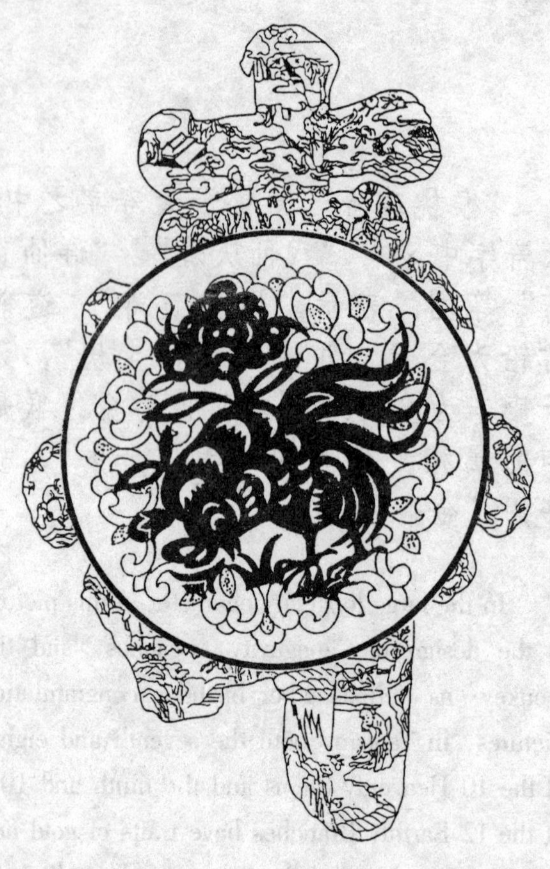

酉鸡贺寿

The rooster congratulates one' s birthday

《花镜》："鸡，一名德禽，……具五德：首顶冠，文也；足博距，武也；见敌能斗，勇也；遇食呼群，仁也；守夜有时，信也。"《春秋运斗枢》："五衡星散为鸡。"雄鸡司晨，守夜有时，故古帝王"以鸡为候"也。

Ancient Chinese literature talks about the five virtues of the rooster: the grace of its cockcomb, the valiance of its sharp claws, its bravery and skill at fighting, its benevolence and habit of signalling others when it finds food, and its faithfulness in keeping watch at night. It is said roosters come from dispersed stars in the sky. As the rooster keeps guard of time, ancient emperors depended on them for keeping the time.

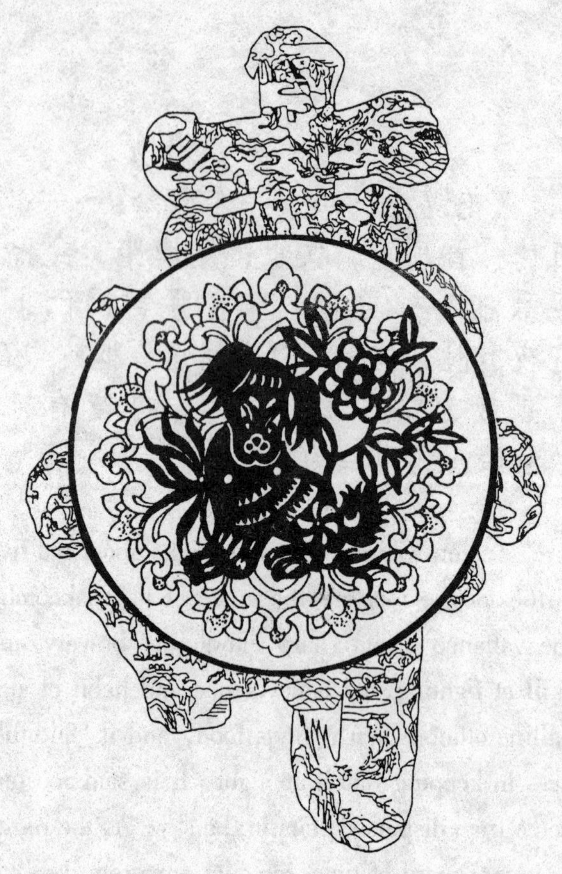

戌狗贺寿

The dog congratulates one's birthday

《七修类稿》：“戌亥，阴敛而潜寂，狗司夜，猪镇静，故狗猪配焉。”古代昼夜十二时，戌时是夜之始，狗守夜，故主戌。在古代正月一日为鸡日，二日为狗日，三日为猪日……有些民族至今仍保留着，以狗为图腾的遗风。

During the 11th and 12th of the Earthly Branches, darkness falls over earth, everything gets quiet as the dog watches over the night. At this time, pigs quieten down, making themselves perfect match with dogs. In ancient China, the first of lunar January is the day of the rooster, the second the day of the dog, and the third the day of the pig. Some minority groups in China still keep the habit of worshipping dogs as their totem.

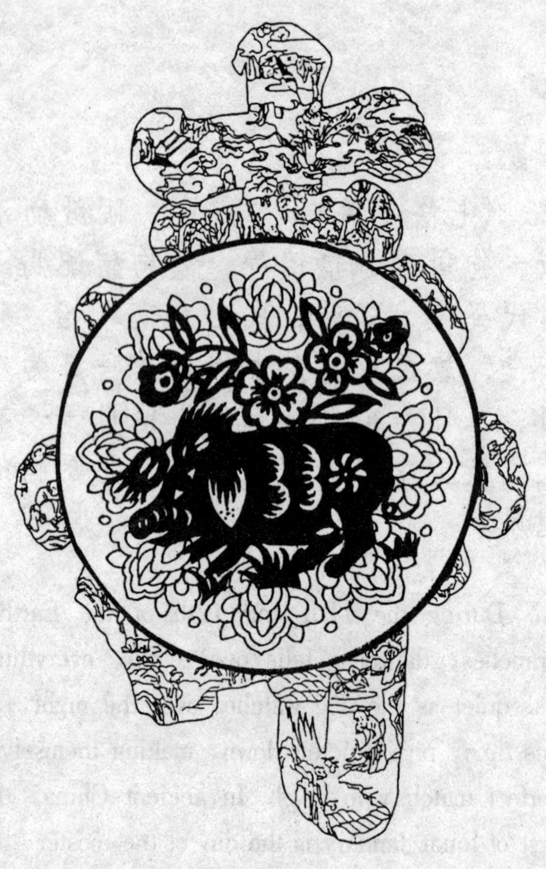

亥猪贺寿

The boar congratulates one's birthday

《说文》："古文亥，亥为豕，与豕同。"《浪迹续读》："观仓颉造字，亥与豕共一笔小殊。""真汞生亥"道教将汞称为木母，故猪又称"木母"。宋太祖赵匡胤生于丁亥，属猪，奉猪为神。猪是最早的家畜，猪亥神也。

The ancient Chinese characters for hai (the 12th of the Earthly Branches) and boar resemble each other very much. Taoism considers boars wood mothers. Zhao Kuangyin, the founder emperor of the Song Dynasty was born in the year of the boar and he worshipped boars as gods. The first domesticated animal, the boar is the god of the hour hai (12th in order).

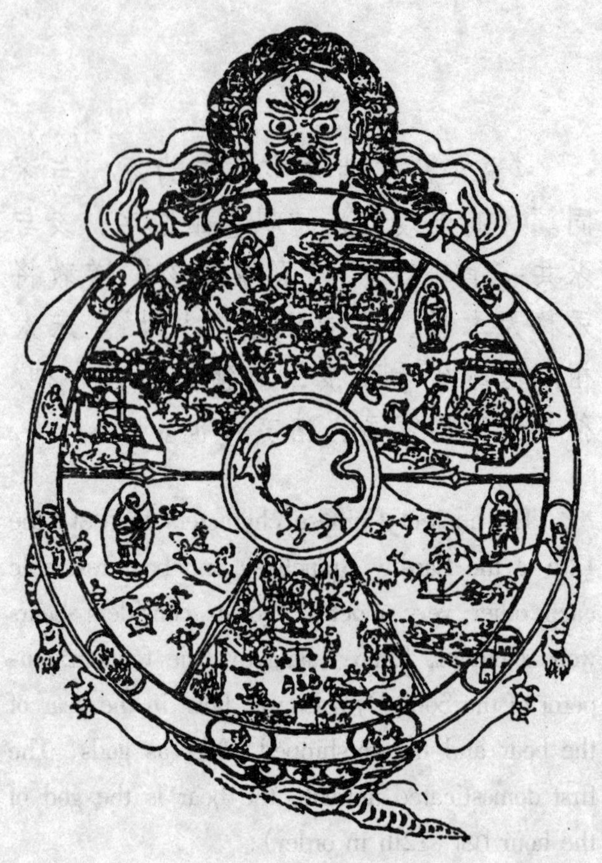

生命之轮

The wheel of life

生命之轮是指人的生死轮回，是藏传佛教喇嘛教劝诫世人去恶从善的符图。佛教认为人死后根据他在世时的功、过、善、恶，再投胎人间时有六种结局：天道、地道、人道、魔道、地狱道、畜生道，即善有善报，恶有恶报。

The wheel of life refers to rotation of life and death, a chart of symbols that Lamaism (Tibetan Buddhism) adopts to persuade and teach people to abandon evil. According to Buddhist, man is subject to six types of results at reincarnation based on the deeds (achievements, mistakes, good and evil) of his life time: he goes to heaven, earth, the world of man, the world of the devil, hell, or beasts. To sum it up, good will be rewarded with good and evil with evil.

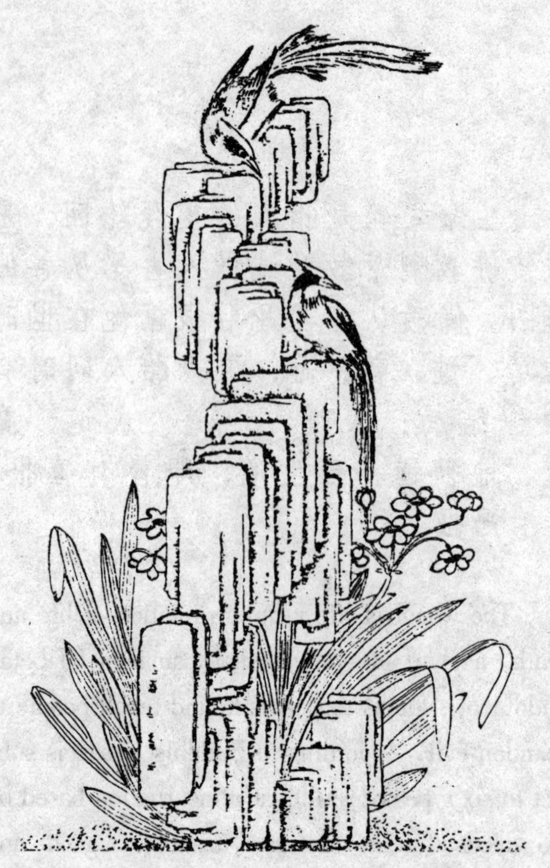

代代寿仙

Longevity and good luck to all generations

绶带鸟即练鹊。雄鸟有羽冠，尾部有两根长羽毛。头部黑色泛蓝光，背部深褐色，腹部白色，美鸟也。图以两只绶带，谐音“代代”。以寿石喻长寿。水仙又称“玉玲珑”、“女史花”、“姚女花”，取其“仙”。形容世世代代长寿吉祥。

Male long-tailed flycatcher has a crest and two long feathers at its tail. Its dark hair at the head has a bluish shine. It is dark brown at the back and white at the belly, a symbol of beauty. The two long-tailed flycatchers mean “generations” as the words are a pun in Chinese. Daffodils are pretty flowers and has the sound “immortal” in it. The message is lasting longevity and good luck.

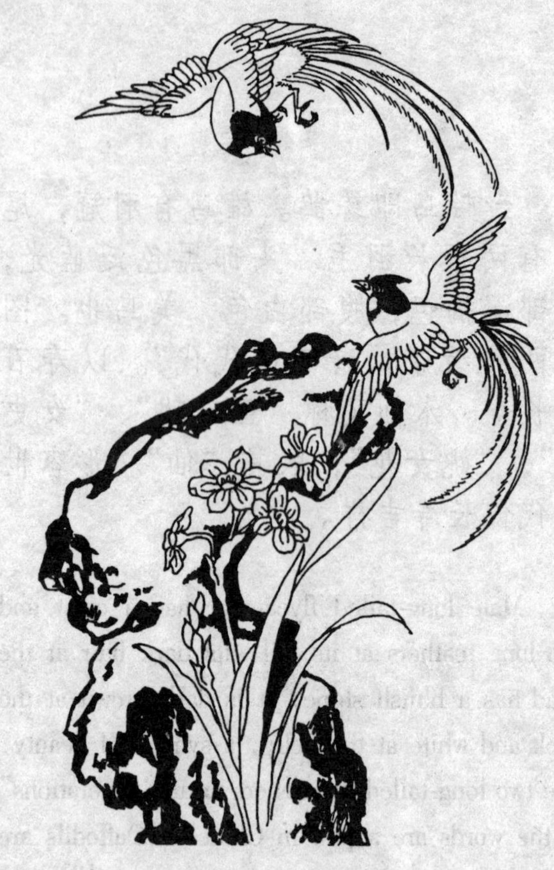

代代寿仙

Longevity and good luck to all generations

《列子·天瑞》："天生万物，唯人为贵。"俗谚："留得青山在，不怕没柴烧。"故"五福"中"唯寿为重"。寿仙是长寿之人，一代长寿，代代长寿是家族最大的福分。图以两只绶带示"代代"，以石示"寿"，以水仙示"仙"。

Ancient Chinese believe man is superior to all creatures on the earth and longevity is cherished by the Chinese more than any other blessings they seek. The biggest fortune of a family is to have not one but all generations of people that enjoy long lives. The two ribbons in the picture indicate generations, the stone symbolizes longevity, and the daffodils immortality.

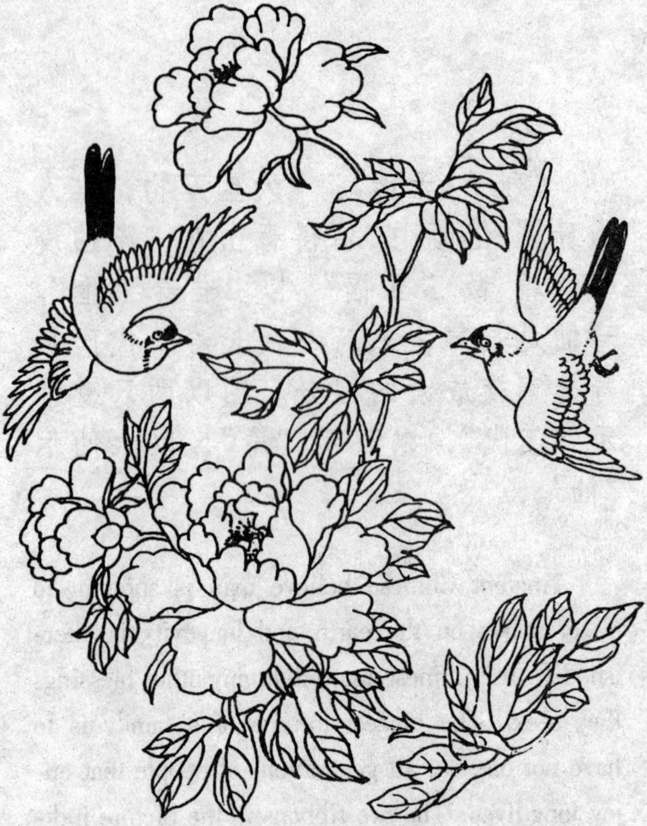

白头富贵

Enjoy a happy life
till white hair appears

白头翁，头顶黑色，眉及枕羽白色，老鸟枕羽更为纯白。旧时也称白发老人为白头翁。白居易诗《重阳上赋白菊》："还似今朝歌酒席，白头翁入少年场。"以牡丹花和白头鸟，寓意夫妇白头到老、生活幸福美满。旧时结婚多用此图案。

Chinese bulbuls are dark at the top of the head but white at the eyebrows and neck. Old bulbuls turn pure white at the neck. White-haired old people were called Chinese bulbuls in the past as indicated in a well-known poem by Bai Juyi. Used commonly for marriage congratulations, pictures of peony flowers and Chinese bulbuls imply devoted spouses enjoy a happy life till white hair appears.

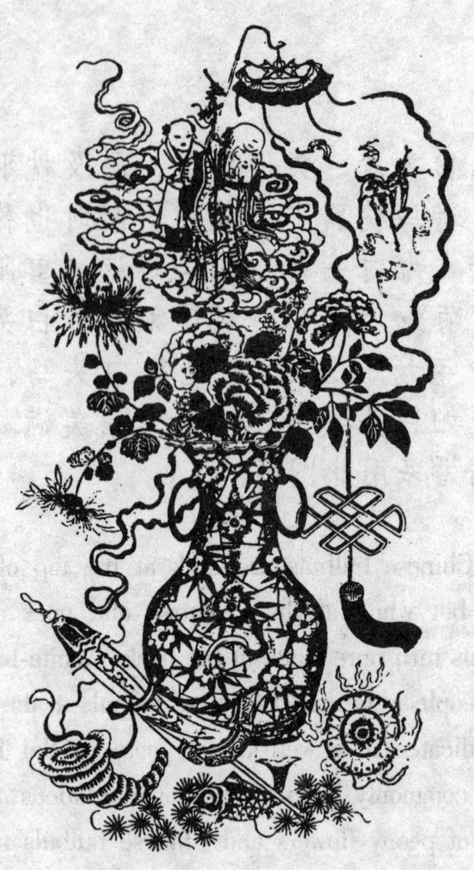

吉祥花瓶

Auspicious vases

这是清代杨柳青的年画，图中集吉祥之大成。瓶中插、绘有象征富贵的牡丹花、桂花等，有喻为四君子的梅、兰、竹、菊等。上有乘祥云而至的福、禄、寿，下有八吉祥。以轮螺伞盖、花罐鱼长，喻绫罗伞盖、华冠羽裳，兆羽化登仙。

This is a New Year picture from Yang Liuing area in the Qing Dynasty. It depicts a gathering of objects related to good luck. Painted on and plugged in the vases are peony (for wealth) and sweet-scented osmanthus (for social rank), plum flowers, orchid, bamboo, and chrythansemums (the four gentlemen). Above these, are good fortune, salary, and longevity on auspicious clouds, and below are the eight auspicious objects. The wheel, spiral shell, umbrella, canopy, flower mug and fish are signs of rising as an immortal.

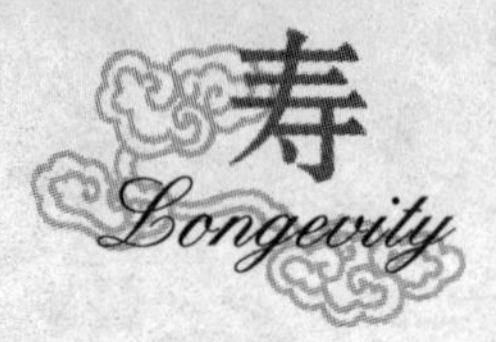

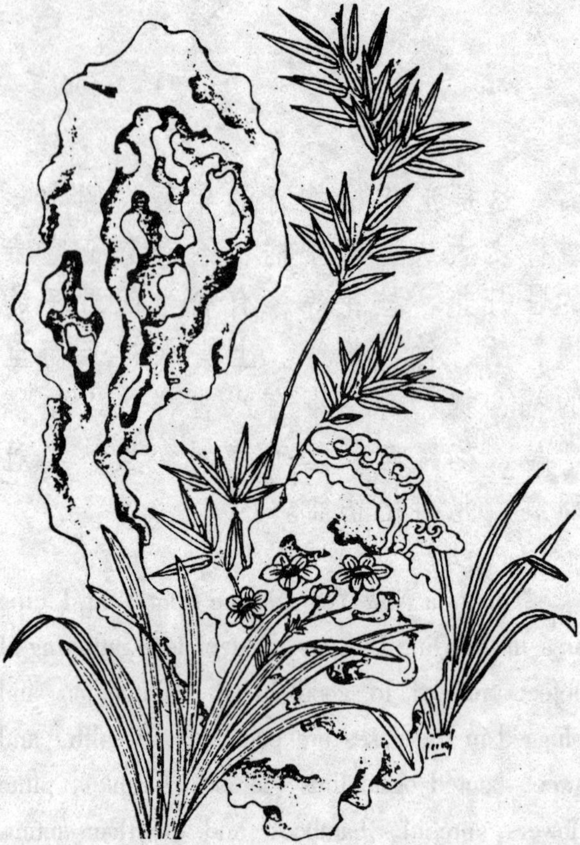

芝仙祝寿

Birthday congratulations from the virtuous

《神农本草》："王者仁慈，则芝草生玉茎紫笋。"灵芝被祝为神物，有驻颜不老、起死回生之妙。水仙花为水中仙子，高洁脱尘，取其"仙"字。竹为君子，四季常青，谐音"祝"。桃取"寿"意。喻具有美好品德的人给健康长者祝寿。

Ancient Chinese writings on plants state that the glossy ganoderma grows when the rulers are virtuous and benevolent. This plant is hailed a divine plant with magic functions such as keeping one looking young and raising the dead. The daffodils are fairies of the water and symbols of elegance. Bamboo is a gentleman plant and stays green all year round. Peaches in the picture indicate longevity. The plants combine to send the following message: people of good virtues congratulate a healthy elder on his birthday.

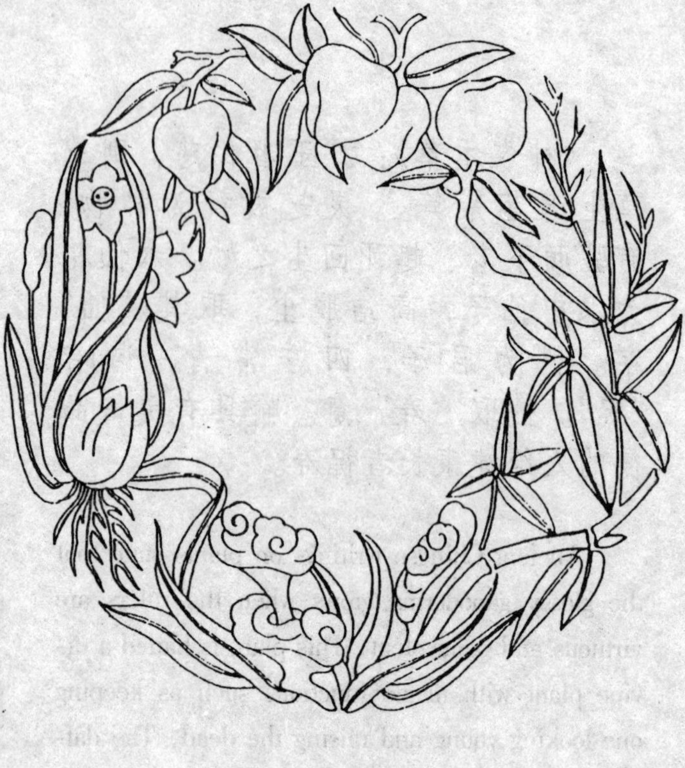

芝仙祝寿

Birthday congratulations from the virtuous

五福以寿为首，五福唯寿为重，故在吉祥图中有关祝颂长寿的内容最多。图中以灵芝示“芝”，以水仙示“仙”，以竹示“祝”，以桃示“寿”，合为“芝仙祝寿。”另外，灵芝、寿桃食之延年，水仙为仙子，竹者常青，均为寿物。

Longevity is the first and most significant of the five blessings and this explains why many good luck pictures feature longevity. The glossy ganoderma and peaches serve to promise longevity. Daffodils are fairies. These plants together with the evergreen bamboo are all objects related with longevity.

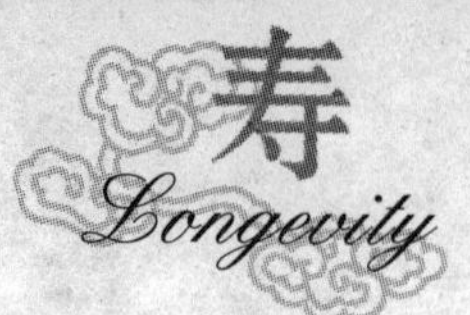

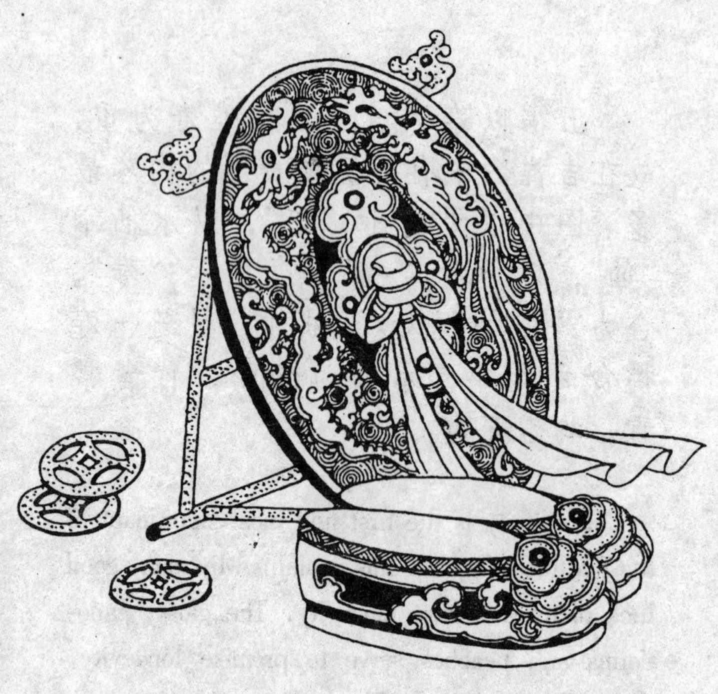

同偕到老

Keep each other's company till old age

我国自商周起，就用青铜磨光制镜。到战国时已很流行，汉、唐时制作更加精美，图中铜镜背面雕有龙凤呈祥纹。左、右两只鞋寓男、女，夫妻。“铜”与“同”谐音，“鞋”与“偕”谐音，合为“同偕到老”，寓意夫妻恩爱白头偕老。

Starting from the Shang Dynasty, Chinese began to polish bronze to use as mirrors. The technique became popular during the Warring States Period, and refined itself in the Han and Tang dynasties. The back of the mirror in the picture has good luck designs featuring dragon and phoenix. The two shoes indicate man and woman, husband and wife. "Bronze" and "together", "shoe" and "accompany" share the same pronunciation in Chinese. So the message is love of spouses who have gone through life together.

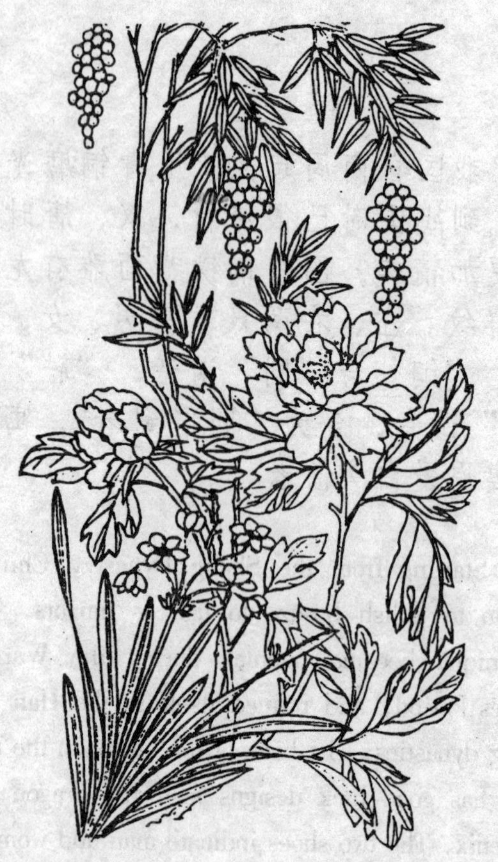

华封三祝

Three wishes from an official

《庄子·天地》："尧观乎华，华封人曰：'嘻，圣人，请祝圣人：使圣人寿……使圣人富……使圣人多男子！'"华封人是在华地守封疆的人。后人多用"华封三祝"祝人多福、多寿、多男子。图以天竹、水仙、牡丹喻之。

According to ancient Chinese literature, the three wishes are longevity, wealth, and many male children. Later the three wishes evolved to be good fortune, longevity, and male children. In the picture, the three blessings are represented by nandina, daffodils, and peony flowers.

多福多壽

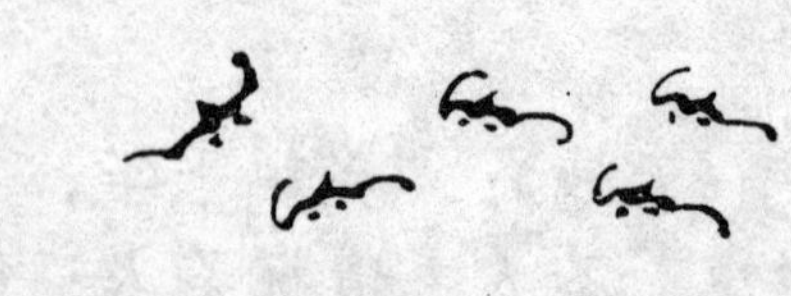

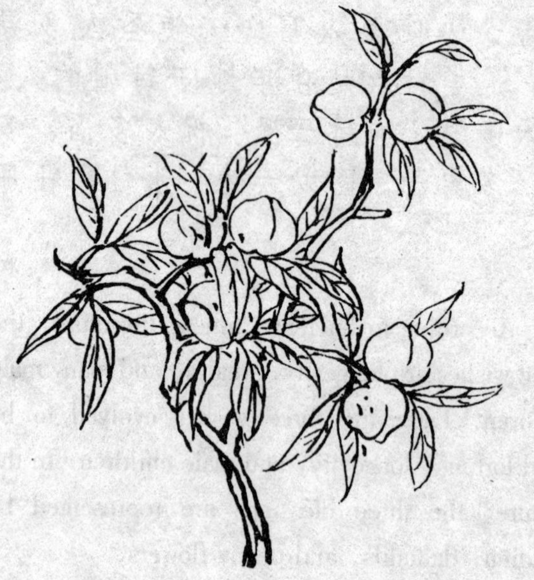

多福多寿

Abundance of good fortune and longevity

福、寿，是最富吉祥含义的两个字。在吉祥图中，蝙蝠、寿桃是喻福、寿的最典型的代表。此类吉祥图也最多，如福寿双全、福寿三多等。多福首推寿，多寿老来福。五只蝙蝠喻“多福”，八枚寿桃喻“多寿”。多福多寿人之大福。

Good fortune and longevity are what good luck is all about. In good luck pictures, bats and birthday peaches are the typical symbols of good fortune and longevity. Most good luck pictures feature good fortune and longevity. Longevity is the most essential good fortune and those who live a long time naturally enjoy good fortune at their old age. The five bats and eight birthday peaches here convey the message of plenty of good fortune and longevity.

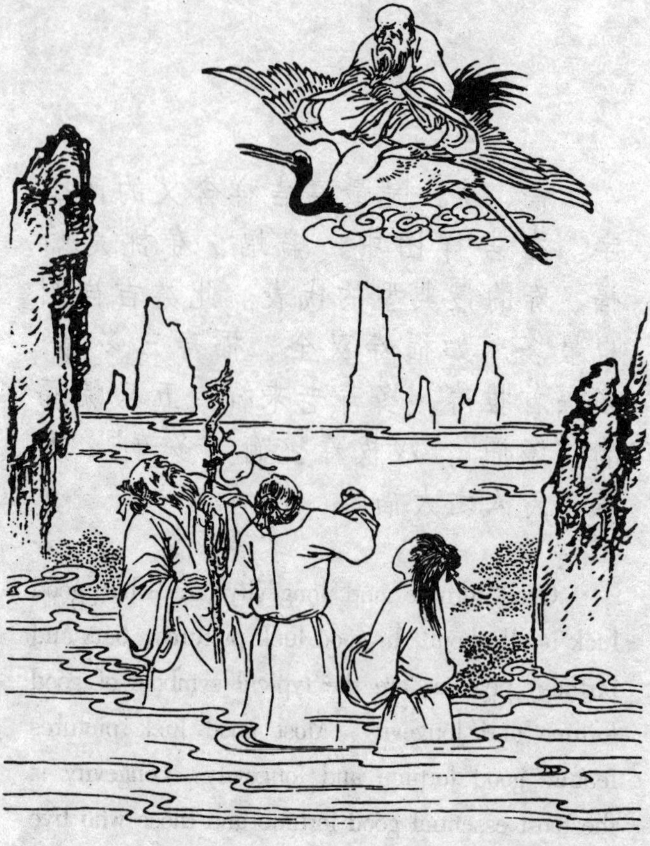

众仙仰寿

The immortals look up to the longevity god

我国早在周秦之时就祭祀寿星。东汉时，仲秋月“祀老人星于国都老人庙”，对古稀老人“授之以玉杖，哺之糜粥。八十、九十，礼有加赐”。尊老之美德自古就有。每逢寿星寿诞之日，乘鹤驾云而至，群仙仰视，颂祝长寿。

Sacrifices were offered to the god of longevity in as early as the Zhou and Qin dynasties. In the Eastern Han Dynasty, on each Mid-Autumn Festival, ceremonies were held to the longevity star. Seventy-year-old elders were given a stick and congee and those in their 80s and 90s received additional gifts. This is the long-cherished traditional Chinese value of respect for the elders. On his birthday, the longevity god would come on a crane and the immortals would look up at him and congratulate him.

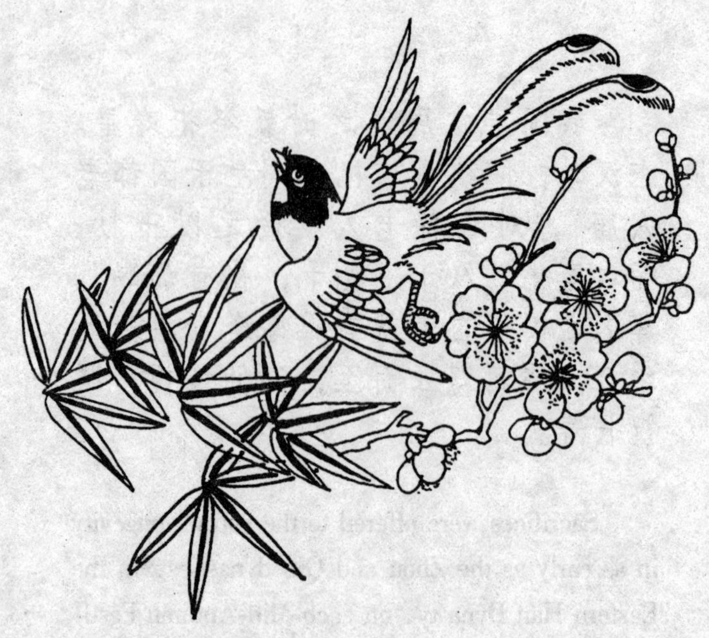

齐眉祝寿

Mutually respectful spouses enjoy long lives

《后汉书·梁鸿传》："为人赁舂，每归，妻为具食不敢于鸿前仰视，举案齐眉。"后来世人称夫妻相敬为"举案齐眉"。"齐眉祝寿"寓意夫妻互敬互爱，白头偕老。图中以"梅"谐音"眉"，以"竹"谐音"祝"，绶带鸟之"绶"谐音"寿"。

A history book from the Han Dynasty tells the following story: a woman was so respectful of her husband that she dared not look at him in the eyes when serving him food. So each time he came back from work, she would lift the board with food on up to her own eyebrows. Later, the phrase "up with the food board to the eyebrows" evolved to be a synonym with mutually respectful spouses. In our picture, the plum flower is a pun with eyebrow, the Chinese for long-tailed flycatcher has the sound of "longevity" in it, and bamboo is a pun with congratulations. The message is mutual love and respect between spouses and growing old till white hair appears.

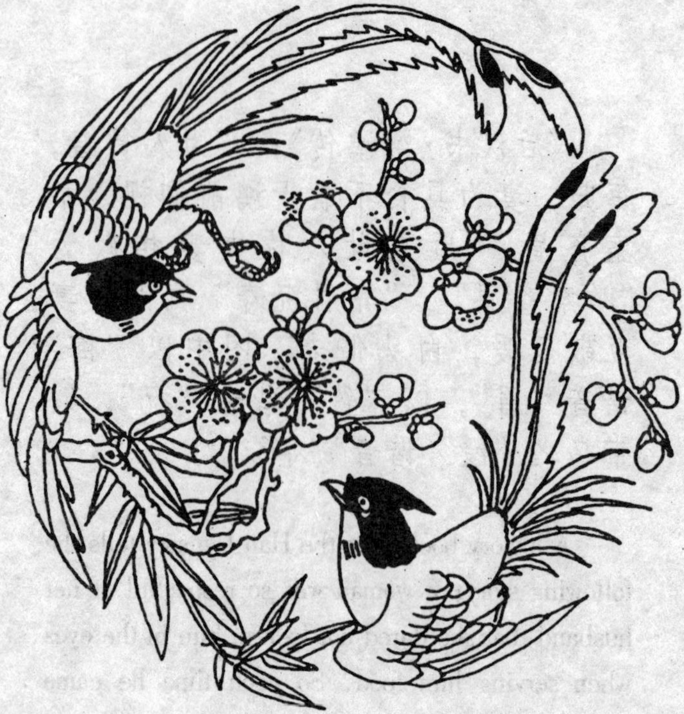

齐眉祝寿

Mutually respectful spouses enjoy long lives

“举案齐眉”以颂夫妻互敬互爱，“齐眉祝寿”以颂夫妻同臻寿域。旧时有喜联：“画眉喜有临川笔，举案欲看德耀妆。”旧时有寿联：“绕膝含饴莱衣竞舞，齐眉举案花甲同周。”“鸿案眉齐礼称曰艾，兕觥手祝诗咏如松”。

While “up with the food board to the eyebrows” is an eulogy for mutual respect between husband and wife, this picture here praises loving spouses that grow to a senior age together. A wedding couplet from the past says: “Gladly the husband draws eyebrows for his wife and her feminine virtue outshines her makeup as she demonstrates great respect for him”. A longevity couplet from the past says: “As the children chew candies and dance round the vines, mutually respectful husband and wife grow to a senior age together”.

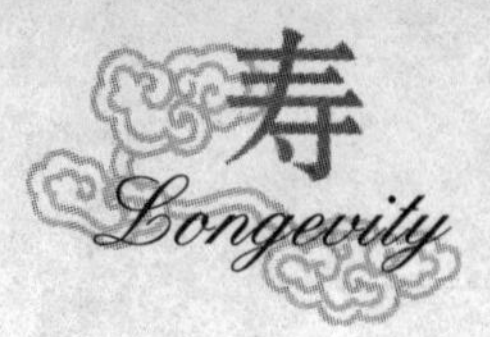

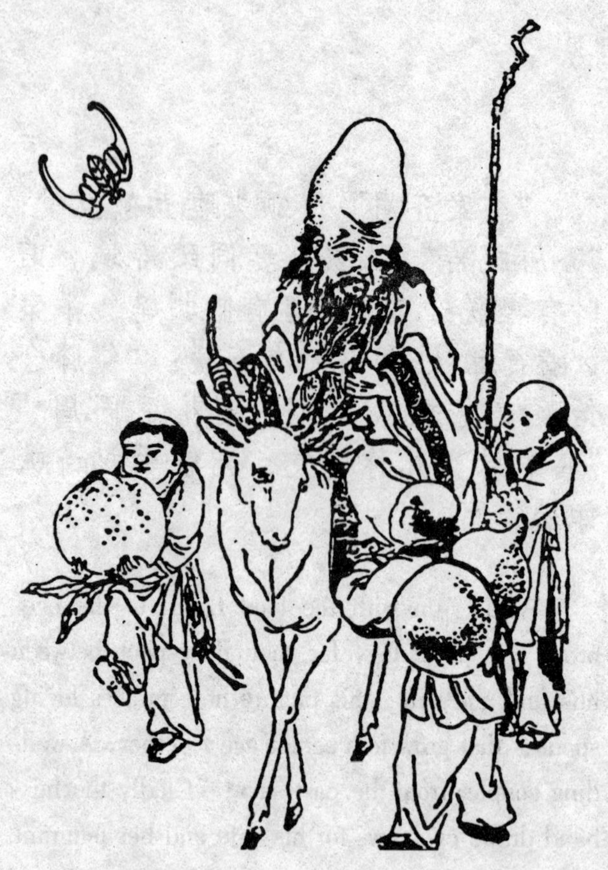

寿比南山

May your age
be as Mountain Nan

《史记·天官书》："老人（星）见，治安；不见，兵起。"老人星司掌国运长短，故历代王朝都将其列入国家祀典。长寿，是人类千古永恒的追求，故寿星备受人们喜爱，旧时有联云："福如东海水长流，寿比南山松不老。"

Ancient Chinese history records state that when the longevity star shows up, the world is in peace and order but if it disappears, violence will break out. The longevity star presides over the fate of the nation and therefore, emperors of all dynasties put him on the list of gods to receive sacrifices. Longevity is the eternal pursuit of mankind and for this reason, the longevity star is a darling among all people. An old couplet from the past reads: "May your age be as Mountain Nan and your happiness as the Eastern Sea".

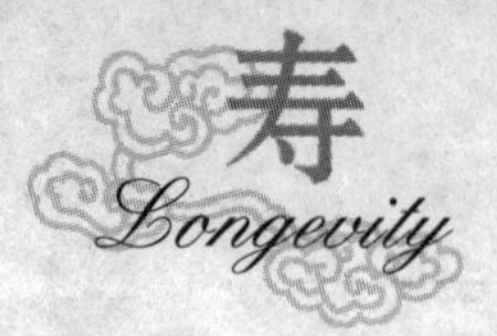

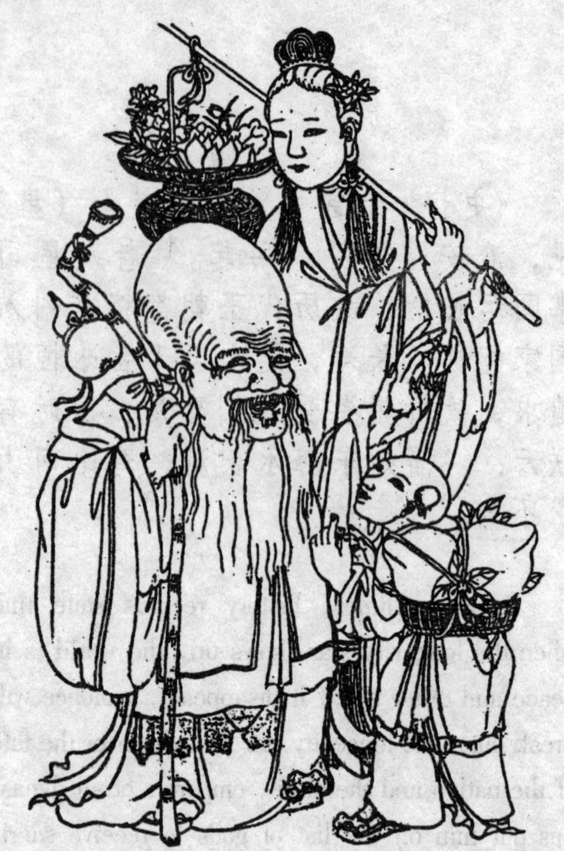

寿星上寿

Celebrating the age of over 100

古代，人有上中下寿之分，100岁称上寿，80岁称中寿，60岁称下寿。旧时有百岁寿幛：“荣登上寿”，“百年人瑞”等。旧时有百岁寿联：“上寿期颐庄椿不老，君子福履洪范斯陈。”60岁以上者过生日可称“庆寿”、“寿星”。

Ancient Chinese considered the age of 100 supreme longevity, the age of 80 medium longevity, and the age of 60 low longevity. Silk birthday sheet and couplet would be presented to those aged 100 with wordings like “congratulations on your birthdays”, “So young looking you are at the age of 100, plentiful are the blessings you have”. Only those over 60 are given grand ceremonies on their birthdays.

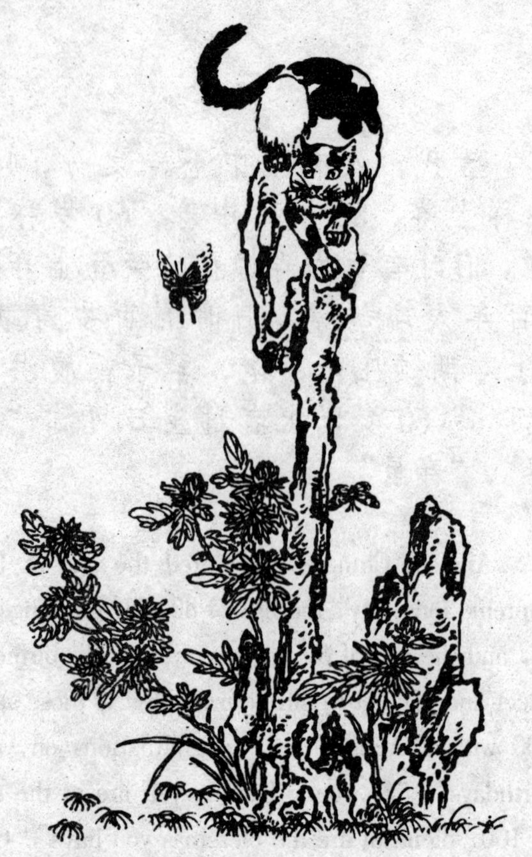

寿居耄耋

To be advanced in years

耄耋指活到八九十岁的老人。人活七十古来稀，活到八九十岁更稀奇。以耄耋之年来形容高寿。图中“猫”与“耄”谐音，“蝶”与“耋”谐音，以“菊”谐“居”，以“寿石”喻“寿”，合为“寿居耄耋”。旧时多作为对长寿老人的赞颂之词。

Maodie in Chinese refers to elders in their 80s and 90s. As not so many people could live to be 70 years of age in the past, those who reached their 80s and 90s were very rare. The cat and butterfly in the picture are puns with “mao” and “die” respectively. Stones imply longevity. This is an eulogy for senior people in the past.

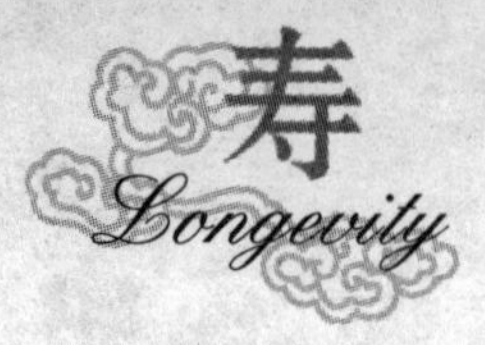

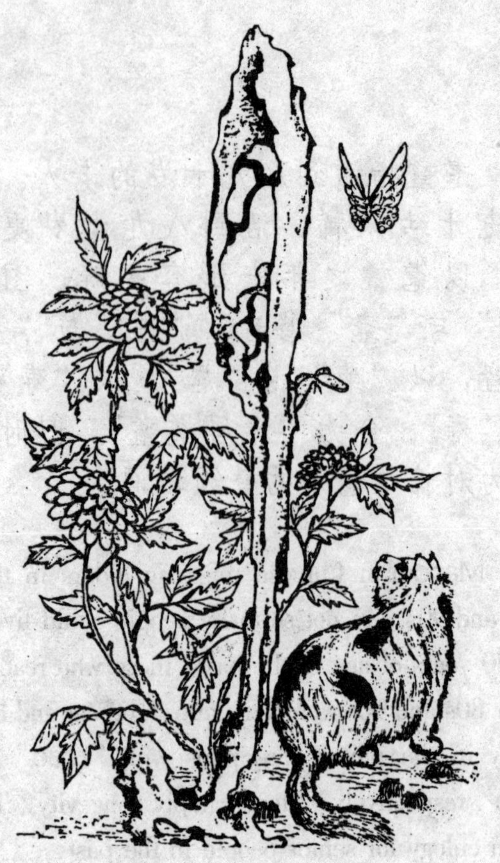

寿居耄耋

To be advanced in years

《礼记》："八十、九十曰耄。"《盐铁论》："七十曰耄。"《毛传》："耋，老也。八十曰耋。"《左传》杜注："七十曰耋。"耄耋泛指年长寿高。"寿居耄耋"可谓长寿，有联："年届耄耋身常健，寿享期颐神更怡。"

Different Chinese history books seem to have some varied interpretation of the word "maodie". To sum it up, maodie in Chinese refers to elders in their 80s and 90s or generally people in their old age. An old couplet says: "Stay healthy and strong though advanced in years; remain happy and self-pleased while enjoying old life".

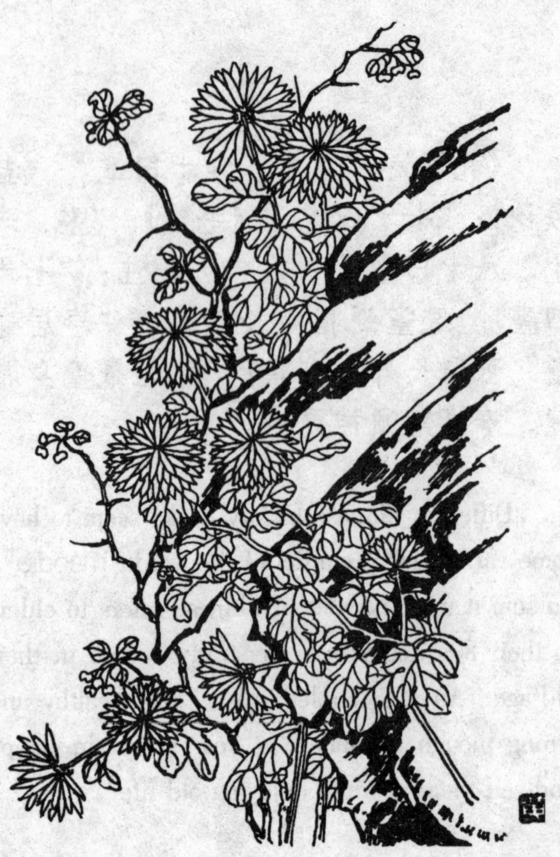

杞菊延年

Enjoy a long life

苏轼《小圃枸杞》："仙人可许我，借杖扶衰疾。"《本草经》云枸杞："服之坚筋骨，轻身耐老。"刘禹锡诗："上品一枝甘露味，还知一勺可延龄。"枸杞自古就被人视作延年益寿的吉祥物。旧时，常以"杞菊"并称，用作祝寿之语。

Ancient Chinese talked about the function of the medlar seeds in poems and other writings: "Given by the immortals, the fruit serves to cure weakness", "the seeds strengthen one's body and lengthen one's life", and "wonderful in taste, the seeds serve to give one long life". The medlar seeds and chrysanthemums are often mentioned together to congratulate birthdays.

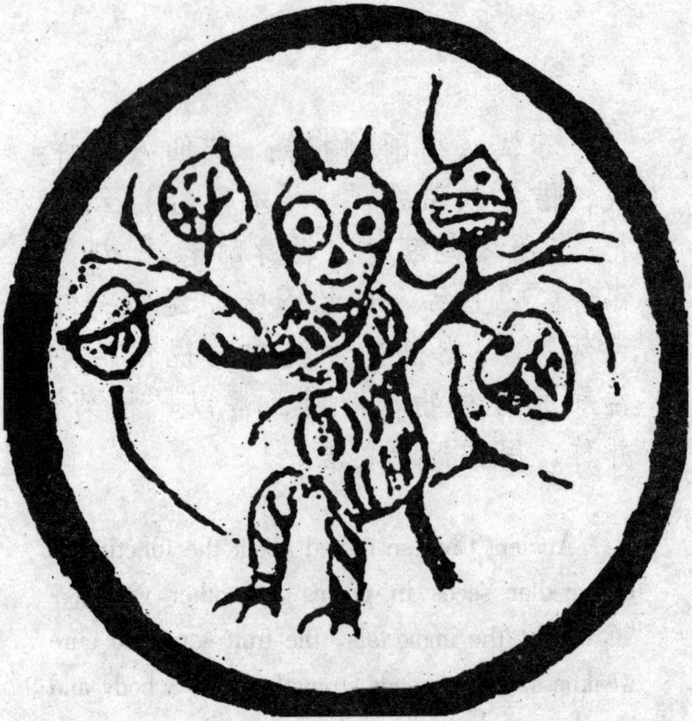

灵猴献寿

The monkey congratulates one's birthday

猴为灵长类动物，在动物中最灵，也与人最似。在民间更被神化为七十二变的美猴王、齐天大圣。在《西游记》中，有美猴王偷吃寿桃之说。“猴”与“侯”谐音，桃有“仙桃”、“寿桃”之称。“灵猴献寿”意为加官进爵，长寿千年。

The monkey is a primate animal. It is the most intelligent of all animals and bears the closest resemblance to man. In folk tales, it is the Monkey King capable of 72 transformations. The story of the Monkey King stealing birthday peaches is recorded in the novel *Journey to the West*. In Chinese, "monkey" and "marquis" share the same pronunciation and peaches are typical birthday fruit known to have the power of turning one immortal. What the picture here means is to get promoted and live for 1,000 years.

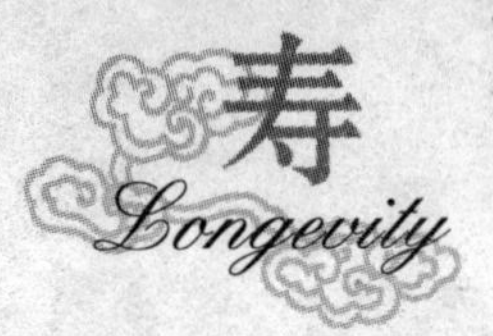

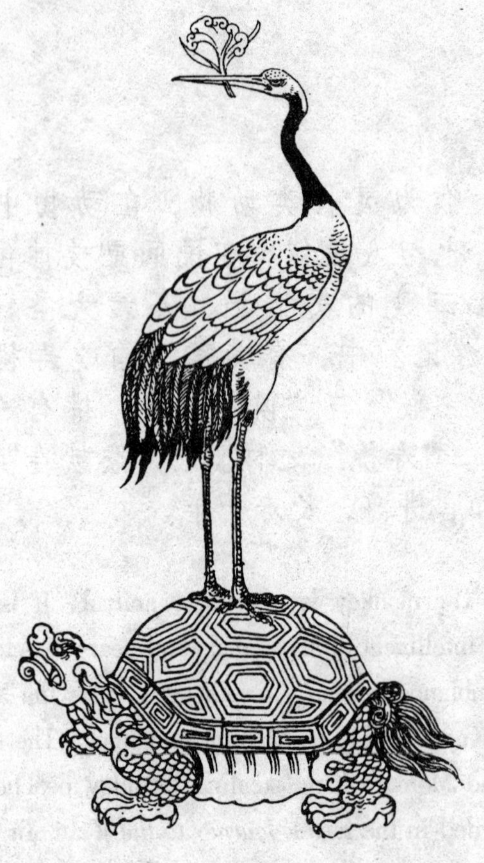

龟鹤齐龄

To enjoy the long life of turtles and cranes

《淮南子》："鹤寿千年，以报其游。"《龟经》："龟一千二百岁，可卜天地终结。"《抱朴子·对俗》："知龟鹤之遐寿，故效其道引以增年。"《游仙诗》："借问蜉蝣辈，宁知龟鹤年。"人与"龟鹤齐龄"，乃高寿也。

Ancient Chinese literature records that turtles and cranes can live up to 1,000 years and a 1200-year-old turtle is capable of predicting the future. Ancient Chinese poets said in their works to "follow the ways of the turtles and cranes to enjoy a long life" and "ask the mayflies if they know about what long lives the turtles and cranes live". Men long to enjoy a long lasting life like the turtle and crane.

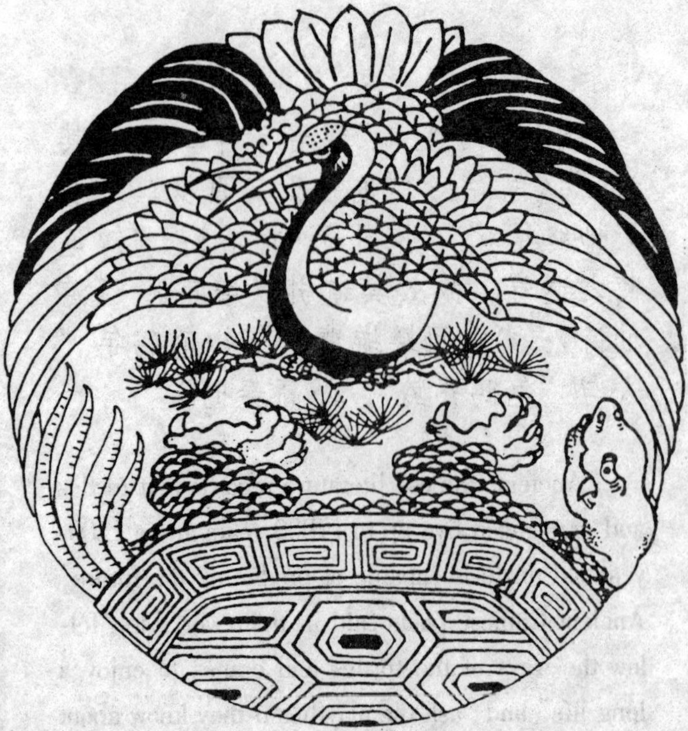

龟龄鹤寿

To enjoy the long life of turtles and cranes

《述异记》：“龟一千年生毛；寿五千岁，谓之神龟；寿万年，曰灵龟，”龟被古人视为长寿的象征物，故以“龟龄”喻高寿。鲍照诗：“龟龄安可护，岱宗限已迫。”鹤为长寿仙禽，故常以“鹤寿”、“鹤龄”等为颂寿之词。

Ancient Chinese writings say that the turtle starts to grow hair at the age of 1000, a 5000-year-old turtle is called a magical turtle and a 10000-year-old turtle a fairy turtle. Turtle symbolizes longevity. A poem on longevity says "how people long to seek for the long life of turtles and Mountain Tai". The crane is a fairy bird and enjoys a long life. The turtle and the crane are also mentioned together in eulogies on birthdays.

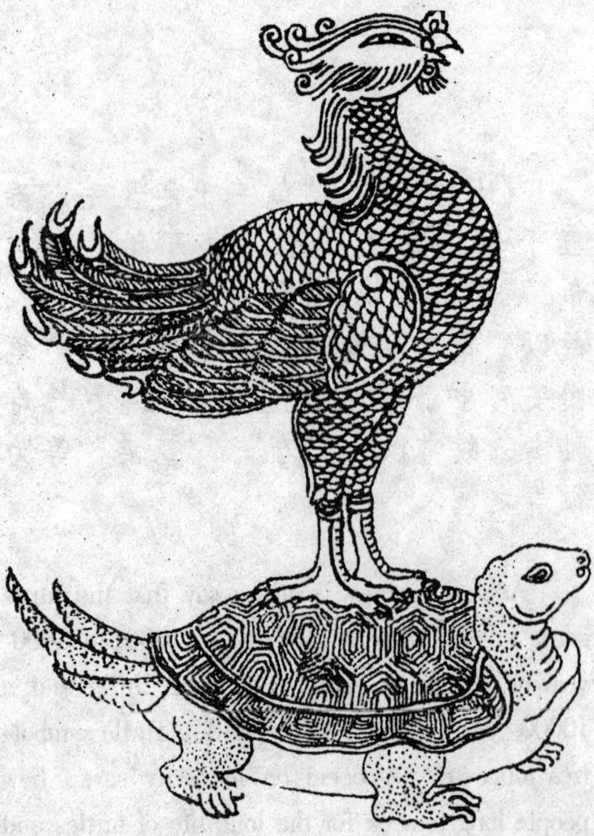

龟凤齐龄

To enjoy the long life of a turtle and phoenix

《大戴礼·易本命》：“有羽之虫三百六十而凤凰为之长。”凤凰是瑞鸟、百鸟之王。在中国的龙凤文化中，龙、凤图案曾为皇家专用。龟凤齐龄图是晚清的吉祥画，很少见。龟是长寿的象征，凤是女性的代表，以贺女性长寿。

The phoenix is the head of 360 kinds of feathered creatures according to ancient Chinese history. The queen of auspicious birds, phoenix was exclusively used by the royal family in ancient China. Good luck pictures featuring the turtle and phoenix are quite rare and this version was produced in late Qing Dynasty. As turtle represents longevity and phoenix female, the picture serves to wish women a long life.

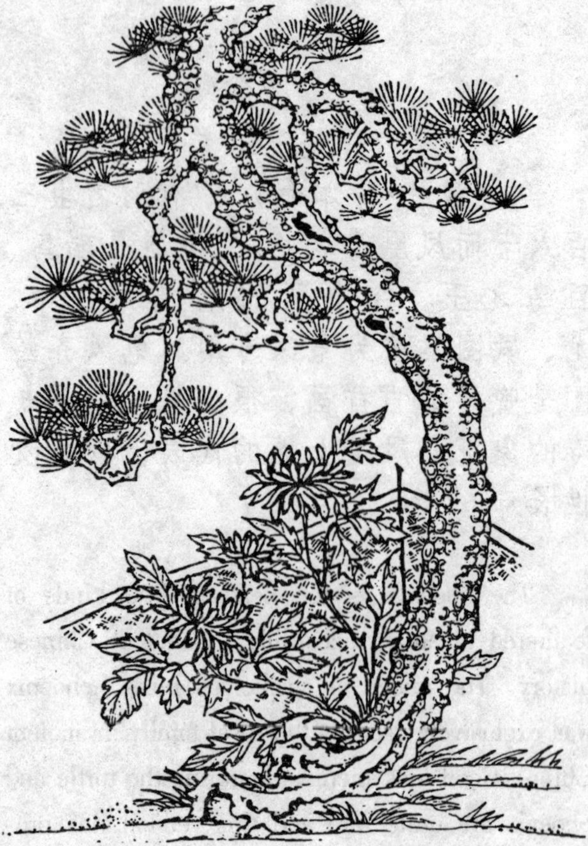

松菊延年

To enjoy the long life of pines and chrysanthemums

东晋·陶渊明《归去来兮辞》："三径就荒，松菊犹存。"也可称为"松菊延年"。松凌寒不凋，四季常青；菊经霜不惧，独吐幽芳。唐·吕温《孟冬蒲津关河亭作》："严冬不肃杀，何以见阳春。"以松菊寓人生虽坎坷，但仍保持高尚品格。

Tao Yuanming of the Eastern Jin Dynasty talked about the long lasting lives of pines and chrysanthemums in one of his poems. The pine does not wither in harsh winter and stays green all year round. Chrysanthemums bloom in frosty weather all alone. Pines and chrysanthemums are often linked with the noble character of those who stay upright in difficulties.

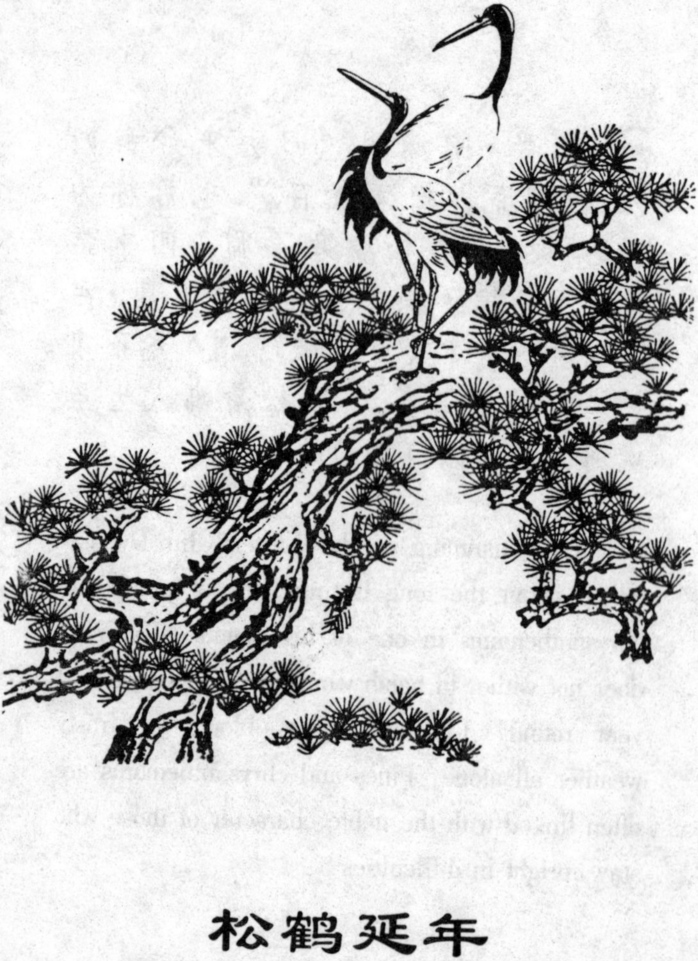

松鹤延年

To enjoy the long life of pines and cranes

延年即延长寿命，《宋书》："今日乐相乐，延年万岁期。"延年即延年益寿，《高唐赋》："九窍通郁，精神察滞，延年益寿千万岁。"旧时祝寿，送松鹤图以求青春永驻。孔子赞松："岁寒，然后知松柏之后凋也。"

The secret to long life has been talked about in ancient Chinese poetry: to be happy and jolly, make sure all parts of the body function properly, and stay in good moods and spirits. In old customs, sending pictures of pines and cranes for birthday celebrations is a common practice to wish people longevity and eternal youth. Confucius made such famous comments on pines: the vitality of pine and cypress trees is self-demonstrative when harsh winter dawns.

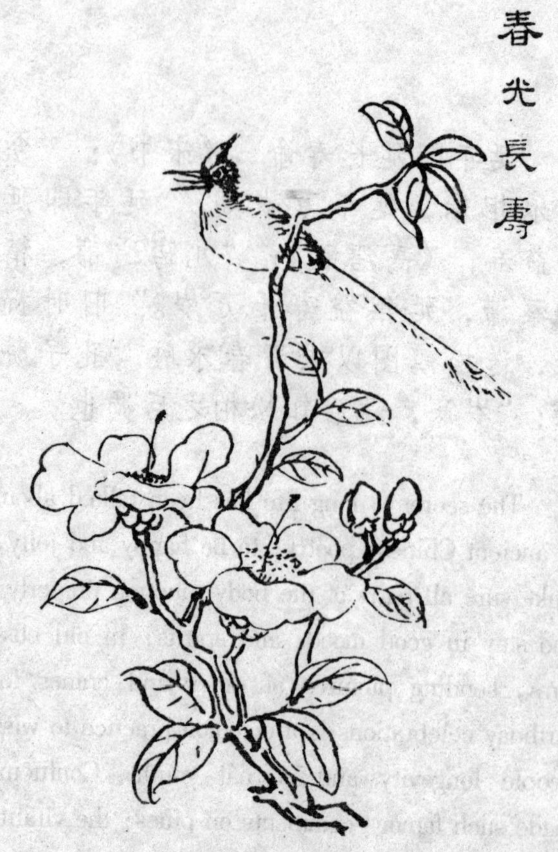

春光长寿

Eternal youth and longevity

曾巩《山茶花》："山茶花开春未归，春归正值花盛时。"《花镜》："山茶一名曼陀罗，……叶似木樨，阔厚而尖长，面深绿，背浅绿，经冬不凋，以叶类茶，故得茶名。"山茶花常被用来表示春意，与绶带相偕，意寓青春不老长寿万年。

A poem about camellia trees goes "camellia flowers start to blossom before spring comes and when spring has come, the flowers are in full bloom". Camellia trees have thick green leaves that highly resemble tea leaves. Camellia is frequently associated with spring. Together with the ribbons (same in pronunciation as "longevity") here, the message is eternal youth and longevity to 10,000 years.

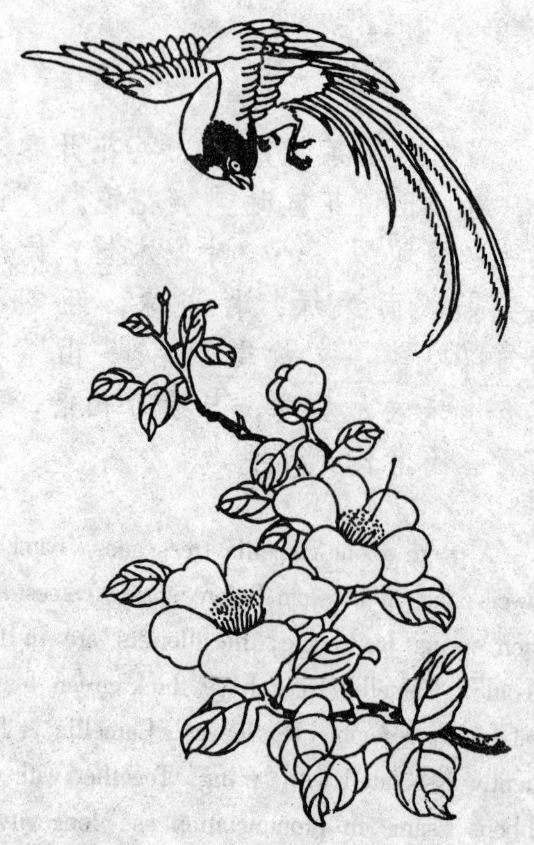

春光长寿

Eternal youth and longevity

宋·梅尧臣《山茶花树子赠李廷老》："南国有嘉树，华若赤玉杯。曾无冬春改，常冒霰雪开。"山茶花耐寒报春，葱郁长青，表示春天。唐·温庭筠诗："海榴开似火，先解报春风。"绶带示"寿"，意为春光永驻，长寿万年。

In a poem by Mei Yaochen of the Song Dynasty, the poet says "A beautiful tree with scarlet flowers grows in the south, and the tree blossoms in spring and snowy winter alike". Camellia trees stand cold weather to announce spring's arrival. Thick in green foliage all year round, the tree is a symbol of spring. The ribbon here indicates longevity. The message is again eternal youth and longevity to 10,000 years.

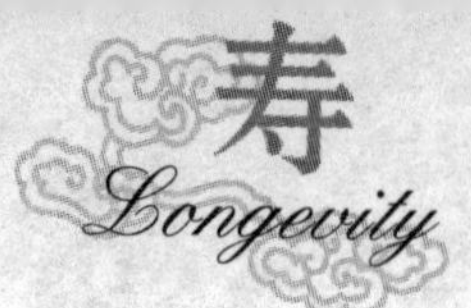

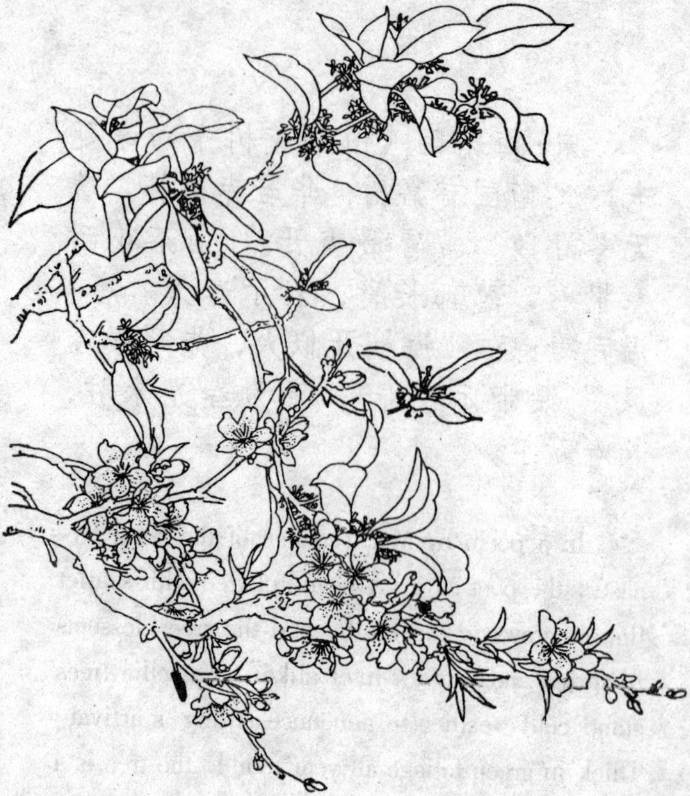

贵寿无极

Wealth and longevity

朱淑贞咏桂诗云："弹压西风擅众芳，十分秋色为伊忙，一枝凌贮书窗下，人与花心各自香。""桂"与"贵"谐音，因而桂花是象征富贵的吉祥物。"桃之夭夭，灼灼其华"。以桃花喻"寿"。"贵寿无极"表达了人们对富贵长寿的追求。

Zhu Shuzhen wrote a poem about the sweet-scented osmanthus tree: "Outstanding among all flowers in the season of autumn is this tree; I pick a twig and place it by the window of my study and feel the harmony of its fragrance with my own mood". The Chinese for the "sweet-scented osmanthus" tree and "wealth" are the same in sound so the tree is seen as an auspicious plant representing wealth. Peach blossoms here represent longevity. The picture embodies aspiration for a long and wealthy life.

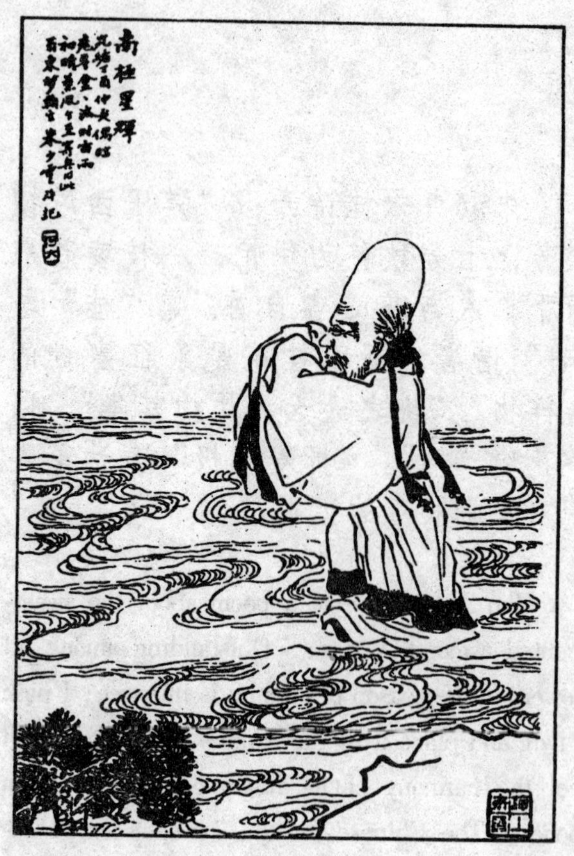

南极星辉

The South Pole Star shines brilliantly

《史记》："狼比地有大星，曰南极老人。老人见，治安；不见，兵起。"《正义》注："老人一星，在弧南，一曰南极，为人主占寿命延长之应。见，国长命，故谓之寿昌，天下安宁；不见，人主忧也。"南极星辉，国昌人寿。

Ancient Chinese history books record that there is a large star, called Old Man of the South Pole. When the star is seen, the society enjoys good order. If it disappears, there will be fighting. It is said that the star can predict the length of life people can live on the earth. Its presence is associated with the prosperity and disaster of the nation. May the South Pole Star shine to bless a prosperous nation and long living people.

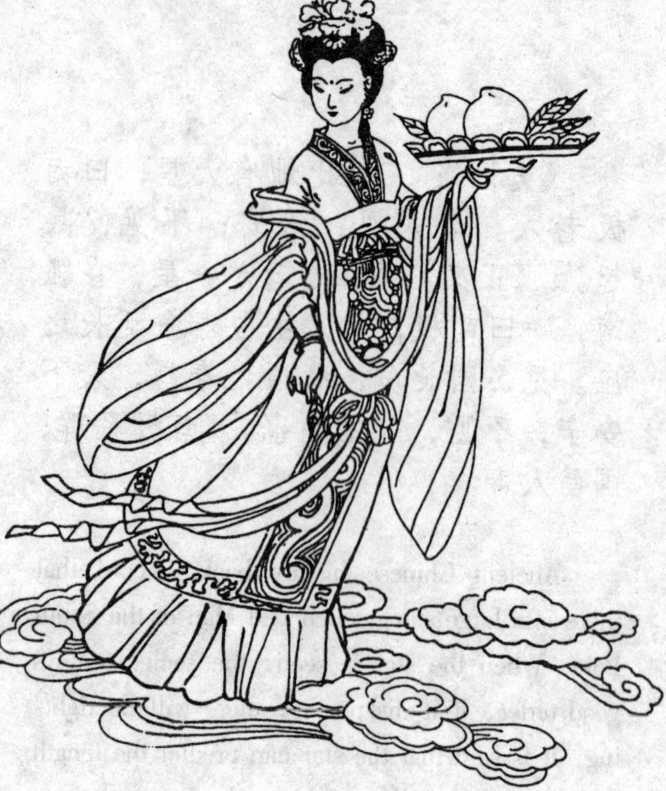

麻姑献寿

Birthday congratulations from Ma Gu

麻姑，是民间传说中的长寿仙女。旧俗每逢妇女祝寿时，常有“麻姑献寿”之图。相传农历三月三日西王母寿辰时，麻姑曾在绛珠河畔以灵芝酿酒献给王母。麻姑生时有道术，能履行水上，还能掷米成丹砂，为仙人王方平之妹。

In folk legends, Ma Gu is a fairy with a long life. Pictures featuring Ma Gu were often pasted when women celebrated birthdays in the past. It is said that each year on lunar March 3rd, the birthday of the Queen Mother of the West, Ma Gu will prepare her wine made from glossy ganoderma at the riverside in heaven. Ma Gu was capable of walking on water during her years on the earth. She was the sister of the immortal Wang Fangping.

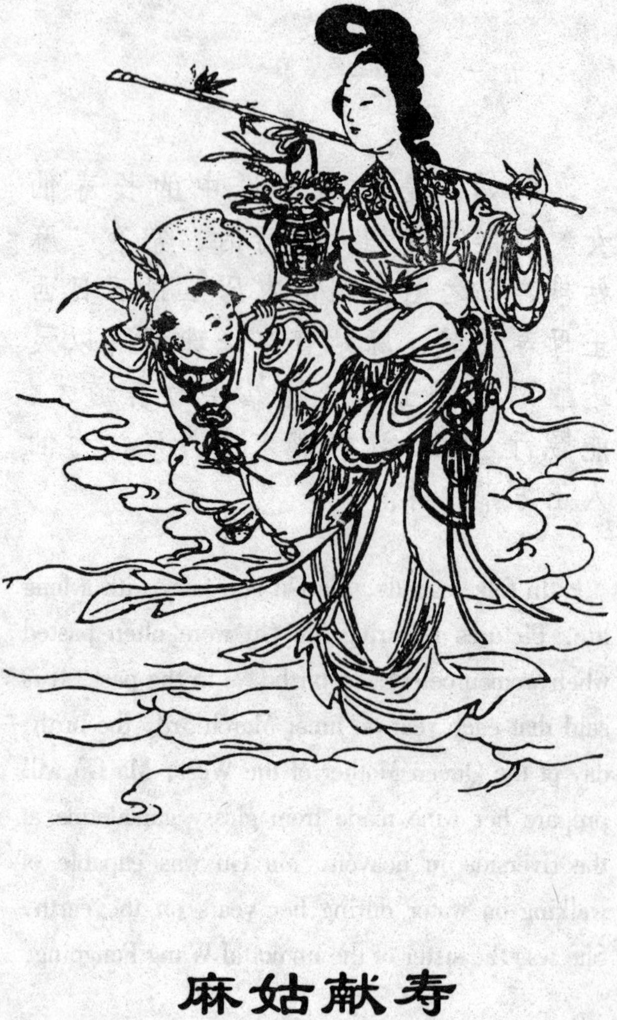

麻姑献寿

Birthday congratulations from Ma Gu

长生不老，长命百岁是人的追求，南极仙翁则是专管长寿的男寿星，而麻姑则是女寿星。旧时妇女祝寿时，多有“麻姑献寿”以字或画的形式出现，做为祝寿的吉利。此图麻姑身旁有一寿桃童子，吉祥图中麻姑常伴南极仙翁。

To have eternal and long-lasting life is the aspiration of all humans. While the South Pole Immortal is the god over longevity, Ma Gu is the goddess. In old times, when women celebrated birthdays, the theme "birthday congratulations from Ma Gu" would appear in writing or picture for good luck. In our picture, a child carrying a peach is standing beside her though Ma Gu is more frequently accompanied by the South Pole Immortal.

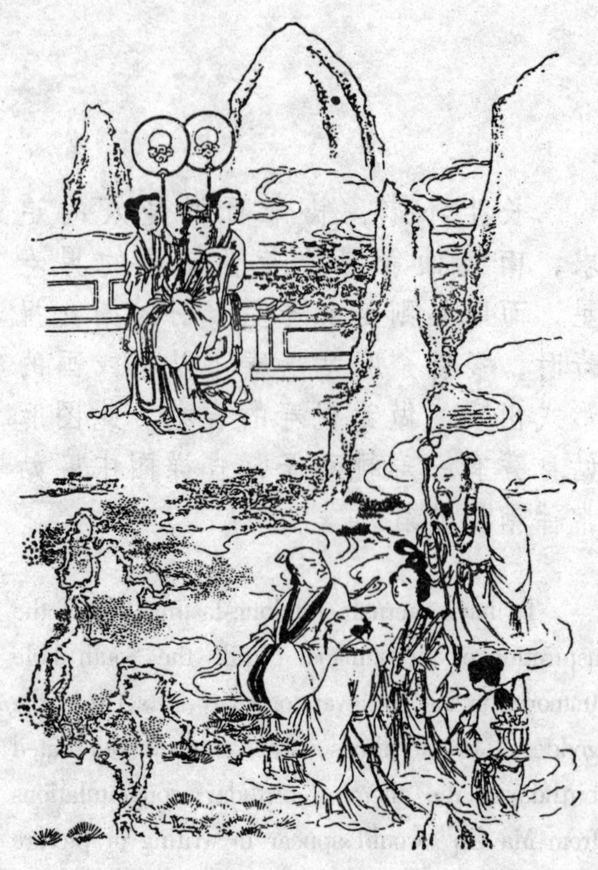

麻姑献寿

Birthday congratulations from Ma Gu

每逢蟠桃盛会，麻姑必与众神仙前往为西王母贺寿。期间有百花、牡丹、芍药、海棠四仙子采摘鲜花，而麻姑则用灵芝在绛珠河畔酿酒，献于王母，以祝长寿。旧时祝女寿有此联句："麻姑酒满杯中绿，王母桃分天上红。"

On the grand flat peach festival, which coincides with the birthday of the Queen Mother of the West, Ma Gu will go to congratulate the Queen Mother together with other immortals. While fairies lily, peony, common peony, and Chinese flowering crabapple pick fresh flowers as gifts, Ma Gu prepares wine of glossy ganoderma at the riverside in heaven. A couplet from the past goes: "As Ma Gu pours her wine into the glass, a light of green shines; as the Queen Mother shares her peaches, the sky has turned red".

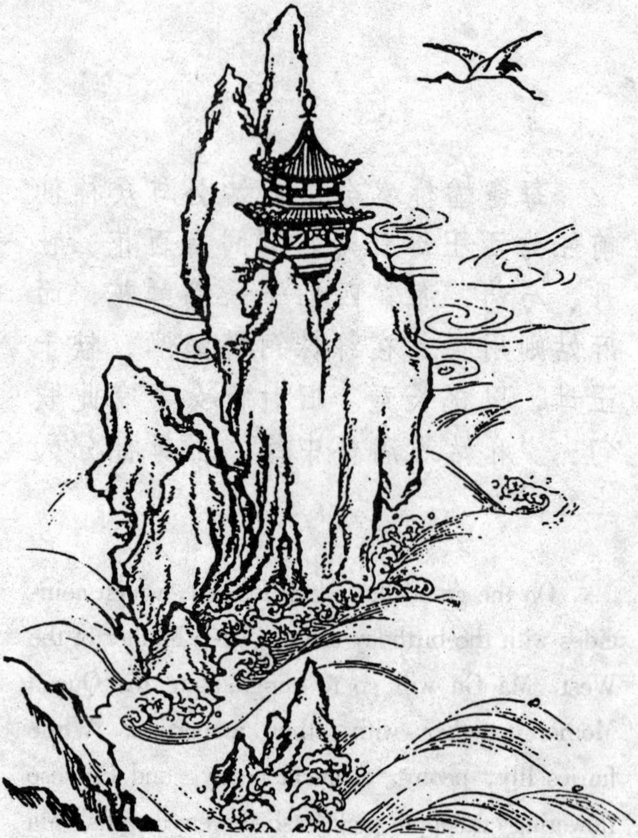

海屋添筹

Chips accumulate at the house by the sea

海屋添筹，常用于形容年寿之增长，图中以海屋飞来寿鹤寓之。《东坡志林》：“尝有三老人相遇，或问之年。一人曰：‘吾年不可记，但忆少时与盘古有旧。’一人曰：‘海水变桑田时，吾辄下一筹，尔来吾筹已满十间屋。’”

The phrase means the addition of years to life. In the picture here, the concept is visualized by a crane that flies over to live in a house at the sea. Ancient Chinese records tell such a story: Three old men met and were asked about their ages. One answered that he could not remember very well but he was an acquaintance of Pan Gu, creator of universe in Chinese mythology. Another said that each time the vast sea turned to farm land, he would put down a chip, and now the chips had filled 10 houses.

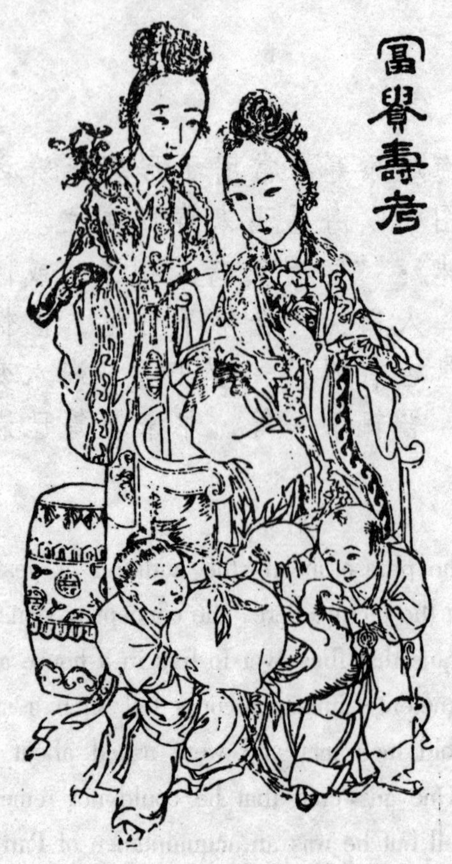

富贵寿考

Wealth and longevity

《诗·大雅·棫朴》："周王寿考，遐不作人。"朱熹集传："文王九十七乃终，故言寿考。"寿考，即长寿。考为老，《新唐书·郭子仪传》："富贵寿考。"图以牡丹示富贵，其中一图以"寿桃"喻"寿考"，另一图以篆书"寿"字喻"寿考"。

Ancient Chinese records tell people that Emperor Wen of the Zhou Dynasty lived for the senior age of 97 years. The Chinese character "kao" stands for "old" and means a long life. As in other good luck pictures, peony represents wealth, and peach longevity.

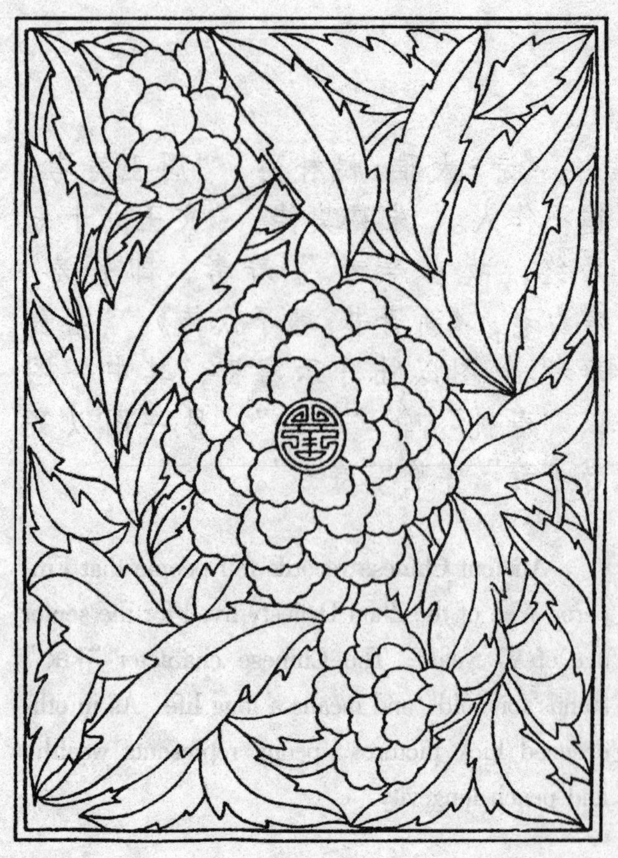

富贵寿考

Wealth and longevity

吉祥图案中心的团寿字，表示长寿，代表“寿考”。而牡丹花图案，则代表“富贵”。周敦颐《爱莲说》：“牡丹，花之富贵者也。”俗谚“有什么别有病，没什么别没钱。”人最怕有病没钱。富有、尊贵、长寿是有福之人。

The round character “longevity” in the center of the good luck picture implies longevity. Peony flowers imply wealth. As the idiom goes, “health and wealth above all else”, one is thrown to hell if visited by poverty and illness at the same time. He who enjoys wealth, status, and longevity has genuine good fortune.

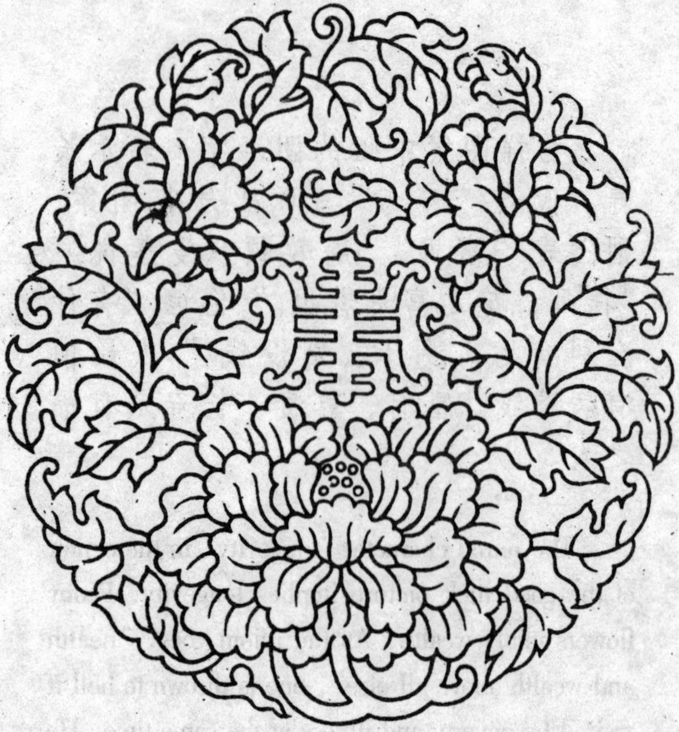

富贵寿考

Wealth and longevity

旧时，许多祝寿的器物上都有“富贵寿考”的图案，以图富贵、长寿之吉利。图中大朵的牡丹吉祥，喜庆。李正封有诗：“国色朝酣酒，天香夜染衣。”“寿考”二字也常入寿联：“颂献嘉平诗歌福祚，人称寿考乐叙纲常。”

The four-character phrase meaning wealth and longevity is on many utensils for birthday celebrations to echo the good luck of wealth, status, and longevity. The large peony flowers add to the festive air of celebration. Li Zhengfeng sang lots of praises to the peony flower: “So astonishingly beautiful is the flower that it resembles drunken beauties in the morning and beats glamorous clothes at night”. Another couplet goes: “Poetry is dedicated to a peaceful society; people in senior age enjoy talking about their families”.

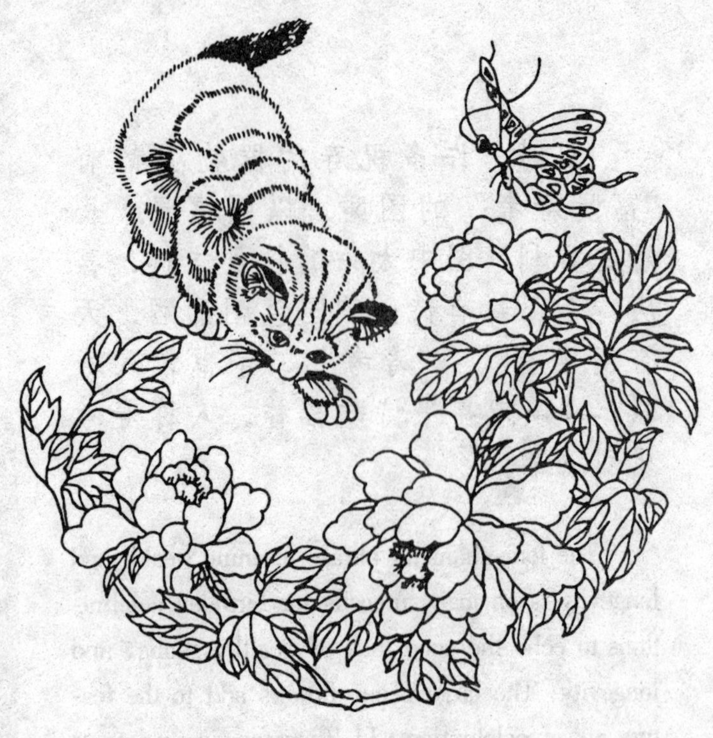

富贵耄耋

Wealth and longevity

《盐铁论·考养》："七十曰耄。"《左传·隐公四年》："老夫耄矣，无能为也。"《毛传》："耋，老也。八十曰耋。"《左传·僖公九年》："以伯舅耋老，加劳，赐一级，天下拜。"牡丹寓"富贵"，猫表"耄"，蝶示"耋"，合为"富贵耄耋。"

Different Chinese history books seem to have some varied interpretation of the word "maodie". To sum it up, maodie in Chinese refers to elders in their 80s and 90s or generally people in their old age. Peony flowers indicate wealth. Cat shares the same pronunciation with "mao" and butterfly "die". So the message is wealth and longevity.

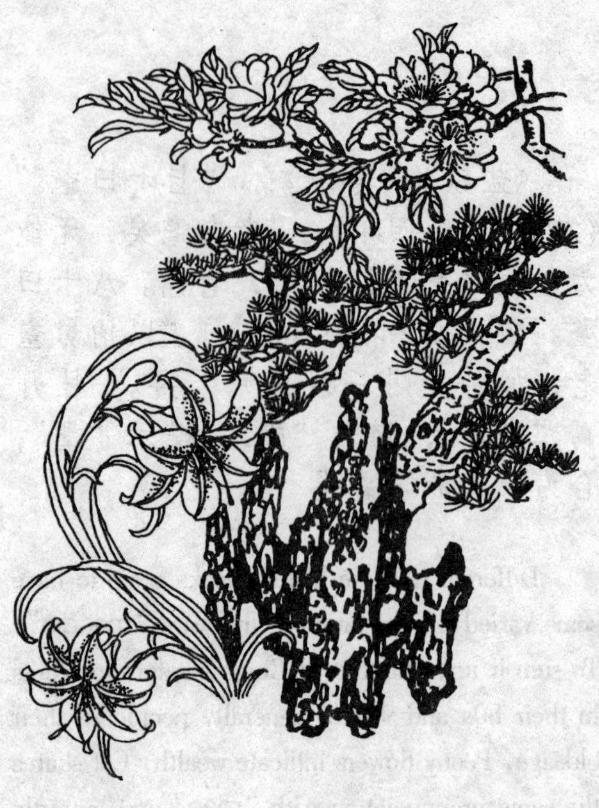

嵩山百寿

Long life like the lofty Mountain Song

麻九畴《送李道人归嵩山》诗云“仰嵩俯嵩，雨濯云烘。”嵩山，古名嵩高，为五岳之中。在河南省登封县北，山上有中岳庙、少林寺等名刹。以嵩山之高，喻人之长寿。图以“松”谐“嵩”，以“石”喻“山”，以“柏”谐“百”，以“桃”喻“寿”，以“萱”代“母”。

Ancient Chinese poems describe the loftiness of Mountain Song: It is soaked in rain water when seen from below and surrounded by clouds when seen from above. Mountain Song is one of the five famous mountains in China. Located in Dengfeng County of Henan Province, the mountain is home to famous temples like the Shaolin Temple. Pine and "song" share the same sound. The stone in the picture represents the mountain, and the peaches longevity.

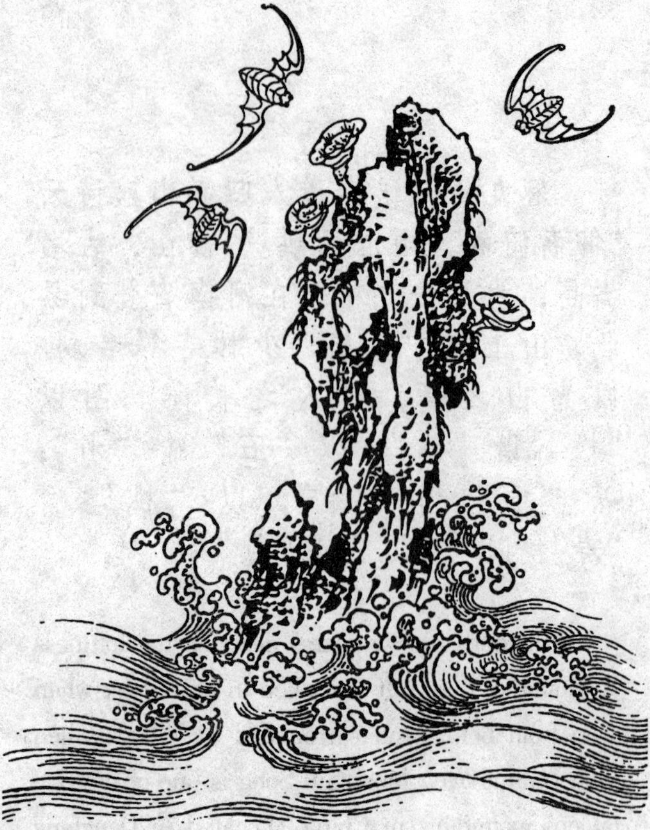

福山寿海

Mountain of good fortune and sea of longevity

福山寿海这一祝寿吉词，与“寿比南山松不老，福如东海水长流。”这一祝寿吉联有异曲同工之妙。图中飞翔的蝙蝠与高耸水中的山石，寓意福山。山石又为寿石，与翻腾的海水，寓意寿海。灵芝作为吉祥物，寓意祝福、长寿。

The phrase conveys the same message as “May your age be as the pines on Mountain Nanshan and your good fortune as the flowing Eastern Sea” through different artistic deliberation. The flying bats and soaring mountain stones imply the mountain of good fortune. Stones are linked with longevity and, together with the churning sea water, mean the sea of longevity. Glossy ganoderma is an auspicious plant and implies blessings and longevity.

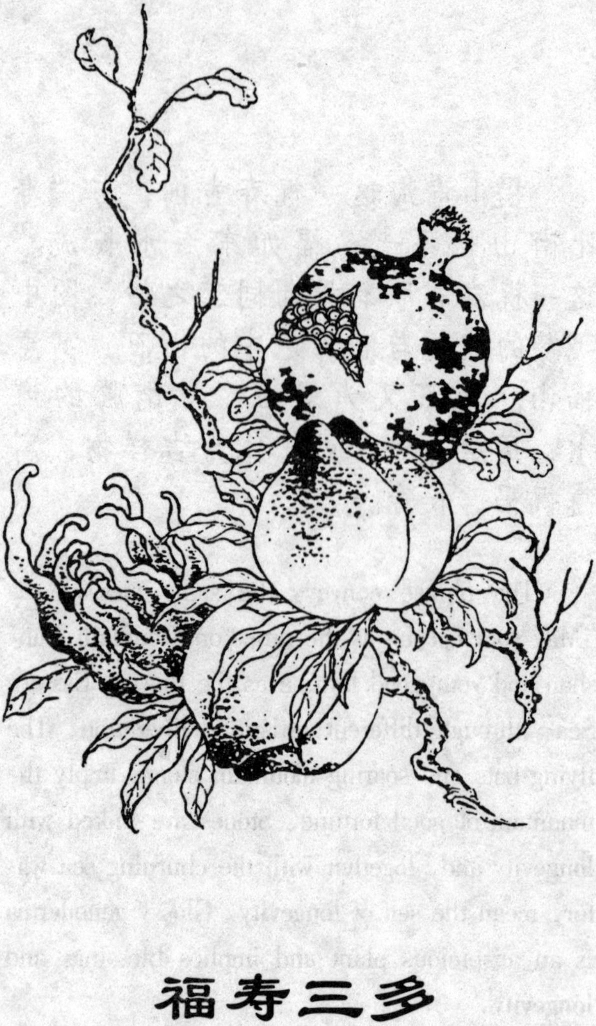

福寿三多

Longevity, lots of wealth and male offsprings

福寿三多，源于华封三祝。《庄子·天地篇》："尧欢乎华，华封人曰：'嘻，圣人，请祝圣人，使圣人寿。'尧曰：'辞'。'使圣人富。'尧曰：'辞'。'使圣人多男子。'尧曰：'辞'。"后多以佛手喻多福，仙桃喻多寿，石榴喻多子。

The three blessings here come from a dialogue between Yao, the ancient emperor, and an official with fief. The official hailed Yao a noble person and wished the emperor to have a long life, lots of wealth and male offsprings. Later, the three blessings have come to be represented by Buddha' s hand, peaches, and pomegranates.

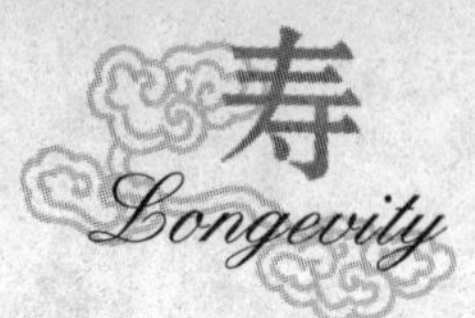

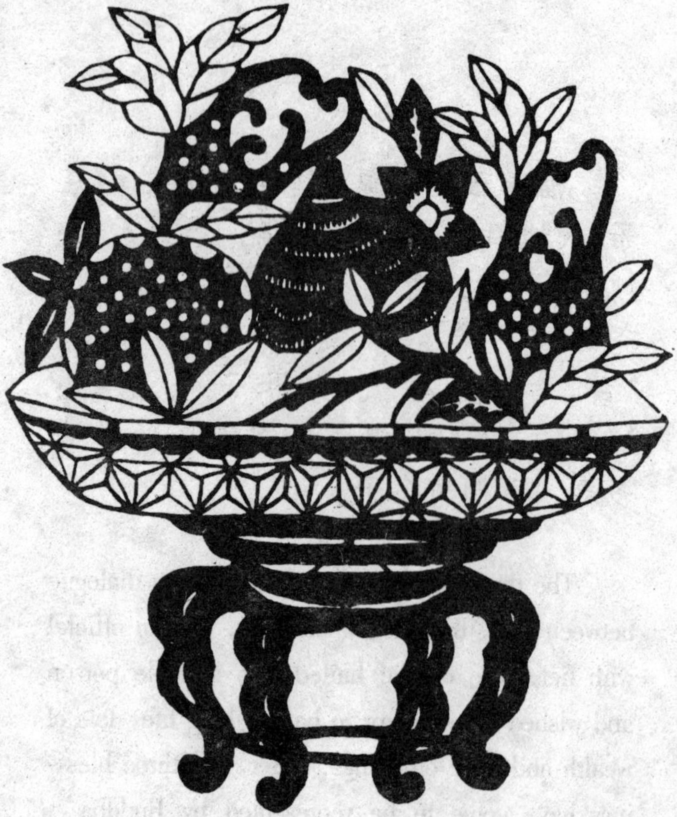

福寿三多

Longevity, lots of wealth and male offsprings

"三多"者，多福、多寿、多男子。图中以果盘中的佛手、寿桃、石榴喻之。佛手原产于印度，形色俱佳，多以之喻佛。又佛手之"佛"与"福"谐音，在吉祥图中多喻"福"。桃为长寿仙果，喻"多寿"。榴为多子之实，喻"多子"。

The three blessings here are good fortune, longevity, and lots of male children represented by the Buddha's hand, peach, and pomegranate in the fruit plate. Buddha's hand originated in India. It has a great shape and bright color and is associated with the Buddha. It is a pun with good fortune and so serves to imply good fortune in good luck pictures. Peaches represent longevity and pomegranate, due to the many seeds it has, implies many children.

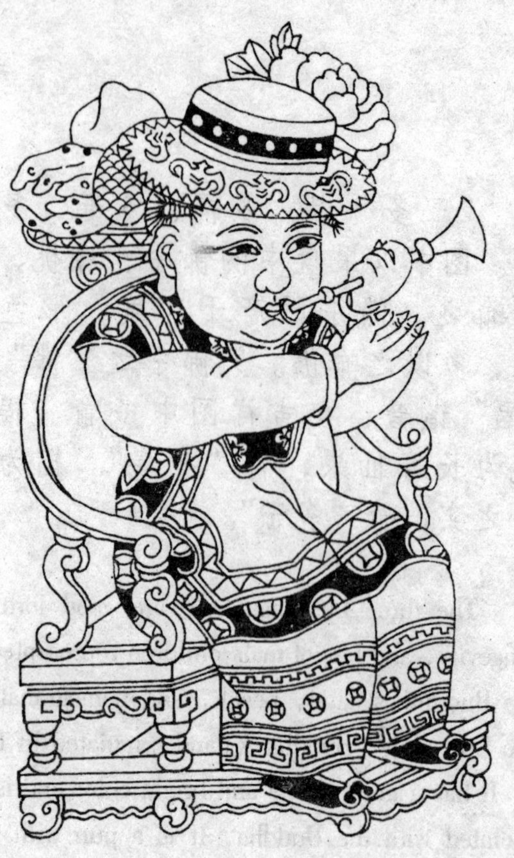

福寿三多

Longevity, lots of wealth and male offsprings

"不孝有三，无后为大"。"三多"中多男子，是旧时家庭中头等重要的事，故图中以一可爱的童子表示"多男子"。图中不仅有佛手、寿桃表示"多福"、"多寿"，而且童子帽子上有蝠蝙图案，衣服上有钱币图案，均有吉祥之意。在吉祥图中，往往集多种吉利于一图。

"Failure to produce offspring is the paramount neglect of one's filial duties". Among the three blessings here, to have male offspring is the top priority in old families. The lovely boy in the picture represents "lots of male offsprings". There is the Buddha's hand and peaches to represent good fortune and longevity. The bats on the hat and the coin print on the clothes of the boy all indicate good luck. Frequently, good luck pictures feature more than one blessing.

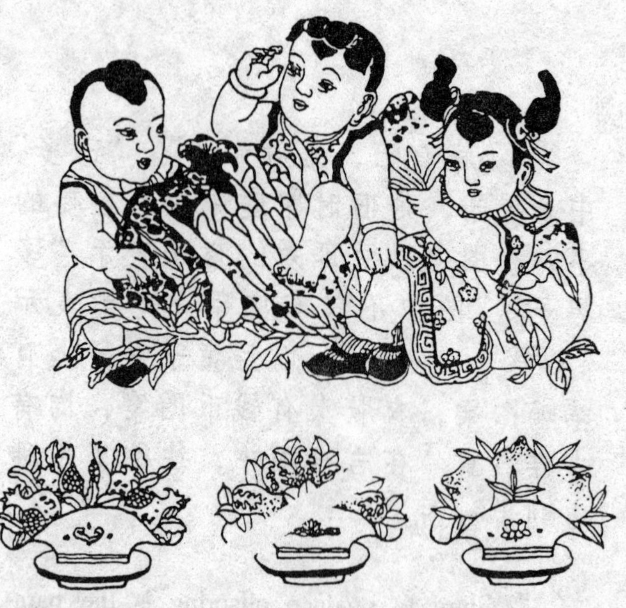

福寿三多

Longevity, lots of wealth and male offsprings

图中以佛手、仙桃、石榴表示"三多",而占据画面主要位置的三位童子,更突出了"多子"之福。旧时有颂金婚诗:"齐眉偕伉俪,饶膝舞儿孙;杖国人弥健,三多萃华门。"还有祝寿联:"华封进三多祝,月恒颂九如歌。"

The Buddha's hand, peaches, and pomegranates in the picture represent longevity, lots of wealth and male offsprings. The three boys in prominent positions emphasize many children. An old couplet from the past praises the life of old couples: devoted and mutually respectful, you enjoy old age while the grandchildren play around you; ever healthy and strong, you harvest blessings in the house.

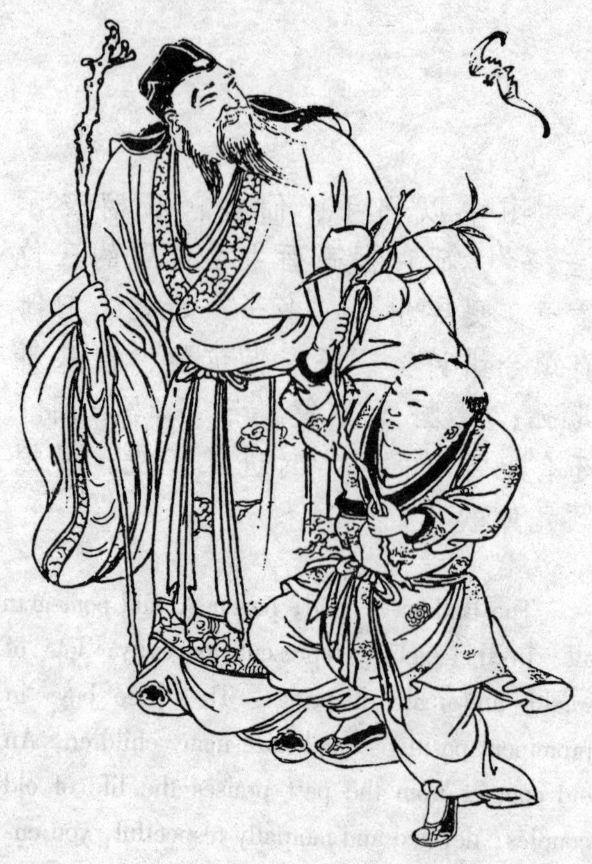

福寿双全

Complete in both good fortune and longevity

福为吉祥之尊，寿乃五福之首。俗话说："福无双至。"福寿双至，那真是双全齐美了，难能可贵。图中的蝙蝠和长寿的老者，分别表示"福"和"寿"。童子双手持一枝寿桃，以童子"双拳"谐音"双全"。另双桃也有福寿双全之意。

Good fortune is the ultimate expression of good luck and longevity the first of the five blessings. A Chinese idiom goes that blessings seldom visit people in pairs. So, to have good fortune and longevity at the same time is truly rare and valuable. The bats and the elder in the picture represent good fortune and longevity respectively. The child holds a birthday peach with both hands, indicating the completeness of two things.

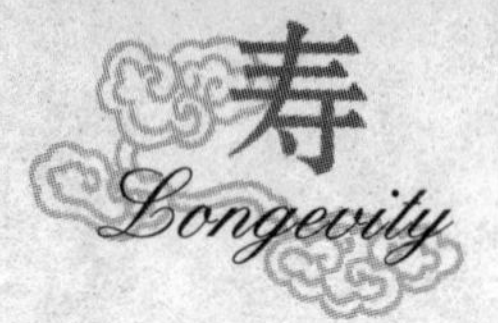

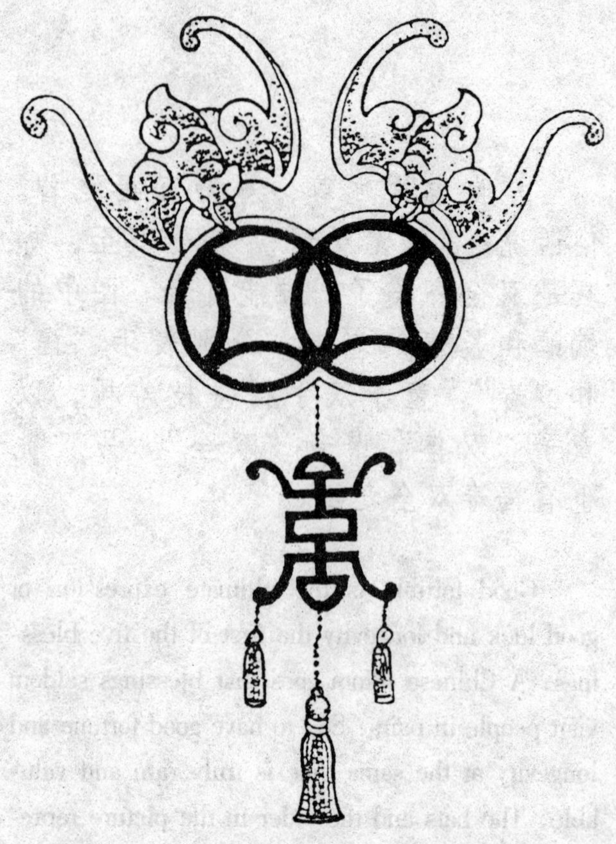

福寿双全

Complete in both good fortune and longevity

福为吉祥之首，寿为五福之尊，福寿双全是人们最大的吉祥。图中的蝙蝠，取其“福”音。寿桃或篆寿字，取其“寿”意。钱古称泉，双钱即双泉，与“双全”谐音，合为“福寿双全”。旧时对有福而又长寿的老人，祝颂福寿双全。

The greatest good luck people can enjoy is to have both good fortune and longevity at the same time. The bats in the picture stand for good fortune. Birthday peaches and the Chinese seal character imply longevity. Double coins refer to completeness in two things. This is an old time eulogy to old people with good fortune.

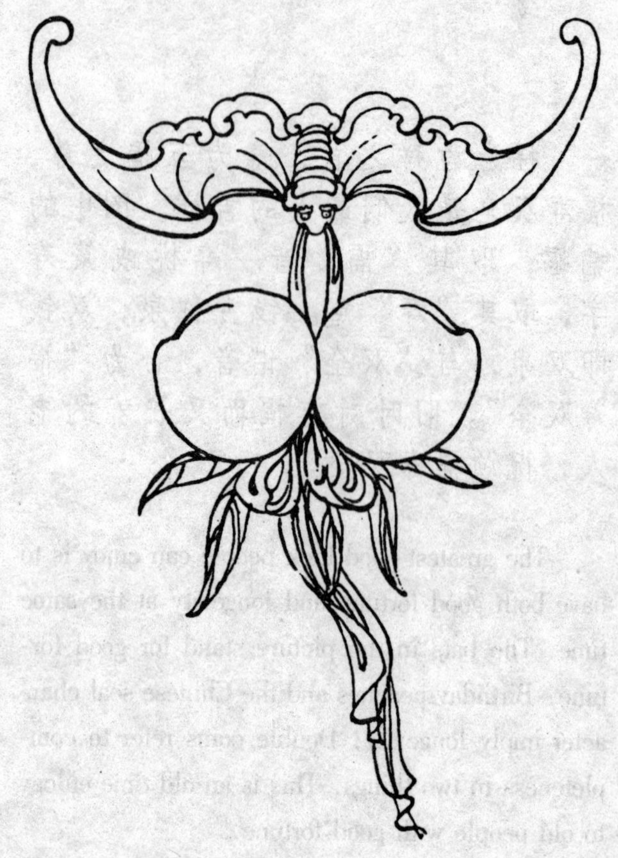

福寿吉祥

Good fortune and longevity

福和寿，是汉字中最为吉祥的两个字，在吉祥图中，蝙蝠和寿桃，是福和寿最经常的代表。吉者福善之事，祥者嘉庆之征。图中以蝙蝠示“福”，以寿桃示“寿”合为福寿吉祥。双桃又有双亲长寿之意，父母长寿，全家吉祥。

Good fortune and longevity are the two luckiest Chinese characters. In good luck pictures, the two are often represented by bats and birthday peaches. Good fortune belongs to those kind at heart and longevity symbolizes a good life. Double peaches also mean longevity to one's parents as the happiness of the parents is the good luck of the whole family.

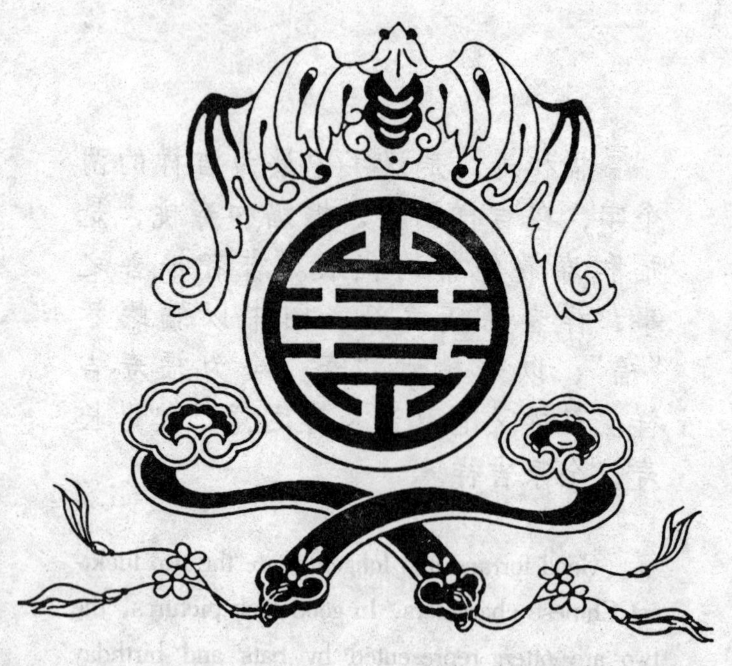

福寿如意

Good fortune, longevity, and to the heart's content

在福、禄、寿、喜、财这“五福”中，以福寿用之最多、最广。在吉祥图中多把“寿”放在中心位置，可见“五福”以寿为首。如意一说是佛具，一说是古之爪杖，后来如意主要指供人赏玩的吉祥物。福寿双全又随人意，乃大福。

Of the five blessings (good fortune, high salary, longevity, happiness, and wealth), good fortune and longevity are the most popular and most talked about. In good luck pictures, longevity is often placed in the center to show its importance. Ruyi meaning as one wishes started as a Buddhist utensil, another story is that it was an itching stick, but later turned to be a good luck object for display and appreciation. What a lucky fate it is to have both good fortune and longevity in addition to having things the way one wishes!

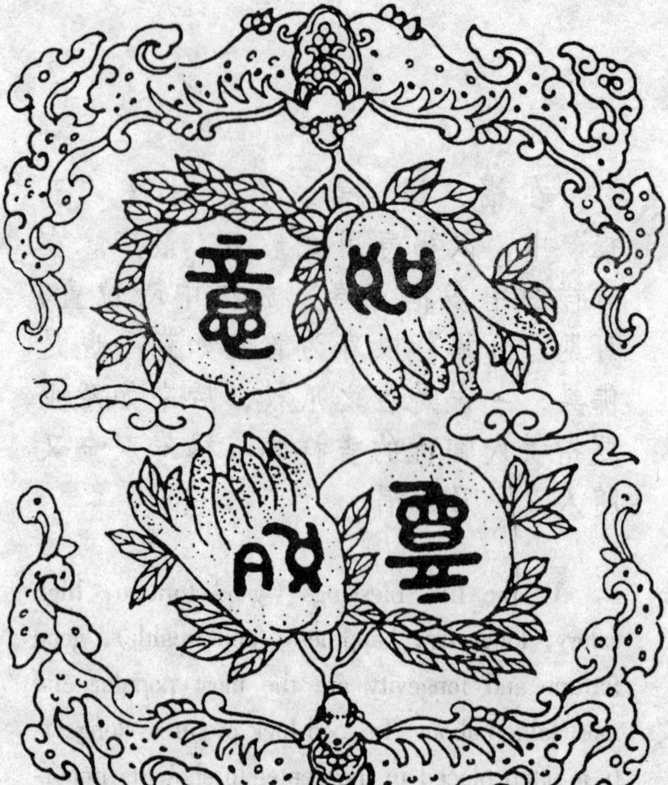

福寿如意

Good fortune, longevity,
and to the heart's content

图中以佛手示“福”，以仙桃示“寿”，与“如意”二字合为“福寿如意”。图中还有蝙蝠和云纹，表示“福运”。即“福寿如意”乃人之“福运”。人的寿命是有限的，富贵又是身外之物，人类对吉祥的追求其实是对生活的热爱。

The Buddha's hand in the picture represents good fortune, and the peaches longevity. Bats and clouds in the picture represent good luck. The number of years man has on the earth is limited and surely wealth has not come with us at birth and can not be taken away at our death. But the pursuit for good luck expresses our love for life.

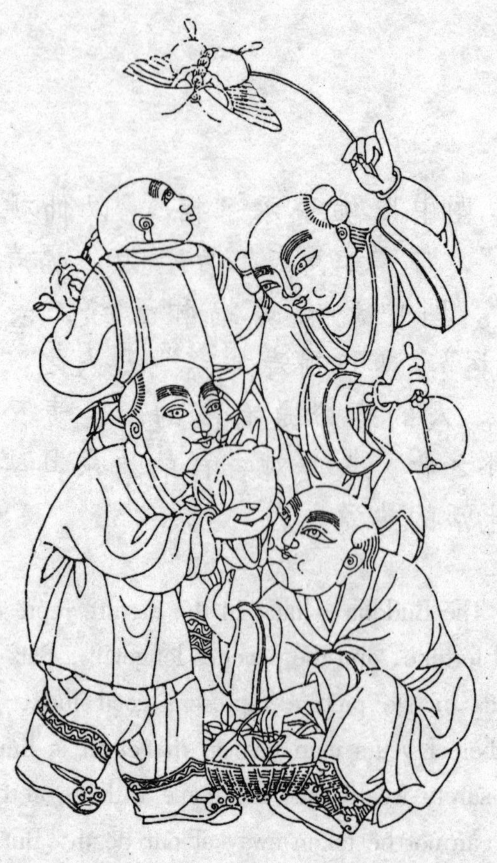

福寿童子

Good fortune, longevity, and children

图为四川绵竹的一幅门画。四位可爱的童子，自含四喜之意。一童子手捧佛手，“佛”与“福”谐音。前面两童子手捧仙桃，表示“寿”。还有一童子手舞蝴蝶，“蝶”与“耋”谐音，耋指年高八十岁，也为“寿”意。年节时福寿童子送来吉祥。

This is a New Year door picture from Mianzhu, Sichuan Province. The four kids indicate four happiness. One kid hold the Buddha's hand implying good fortune. The birthday peaches in the hands of the other two kids at the front refer to longevity. Yet another kid is playing with a butterfly, which also means longevity. At Chinese New Year, the children have sent over good luck to the households.

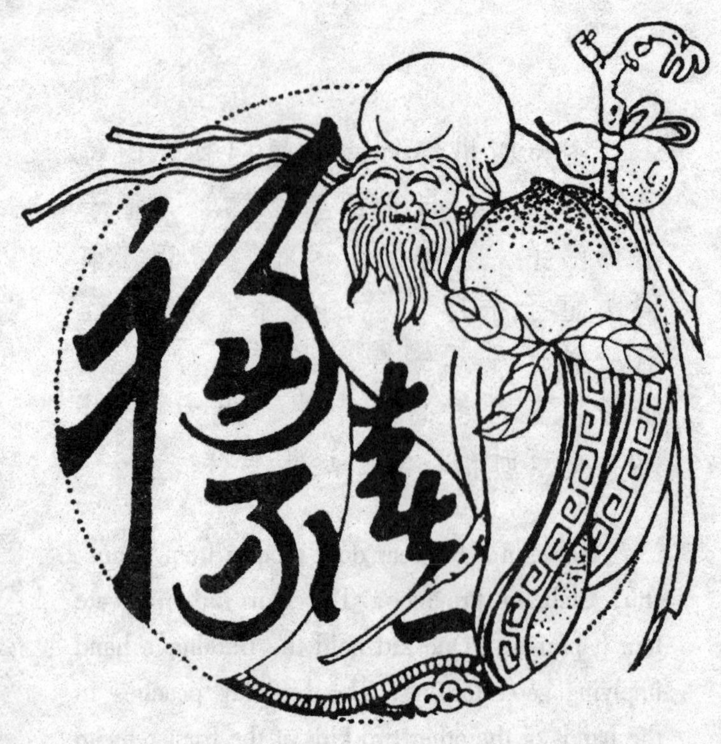

福禄寿喜

Good fortune, salary, longevity, and happiness

宋朝欧阳修《纪德陈情上致政太傅杜相公》诗云："事国一心勤以瘁，还家五福寿而康。"春联中亦有"人臻五福，花满三春"。五福指福、禄、寿、喜、财。在中国传统文化中，对财往往羞于启齿，故有时只提福、禄、寿、喜。

Ouyang Xiu of the Song Dynasty said this in one of his poems about the life of a court official: devoted and diligent in handling state affairs at work and enjoy the five blessings of life at home. Some New Year couplets also mentioned the five blessings: may people enjoy a life full of blessings and let flowers bloom throughout spring time. The five blessings include wealth which people tend to avoid talking due to influence of traditional Chinese culture.

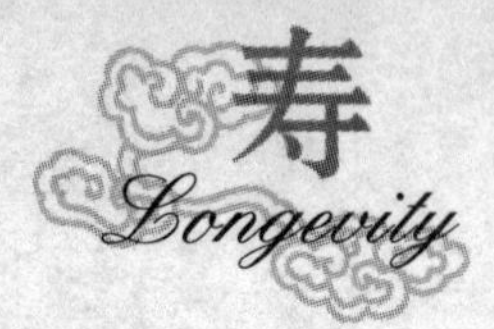

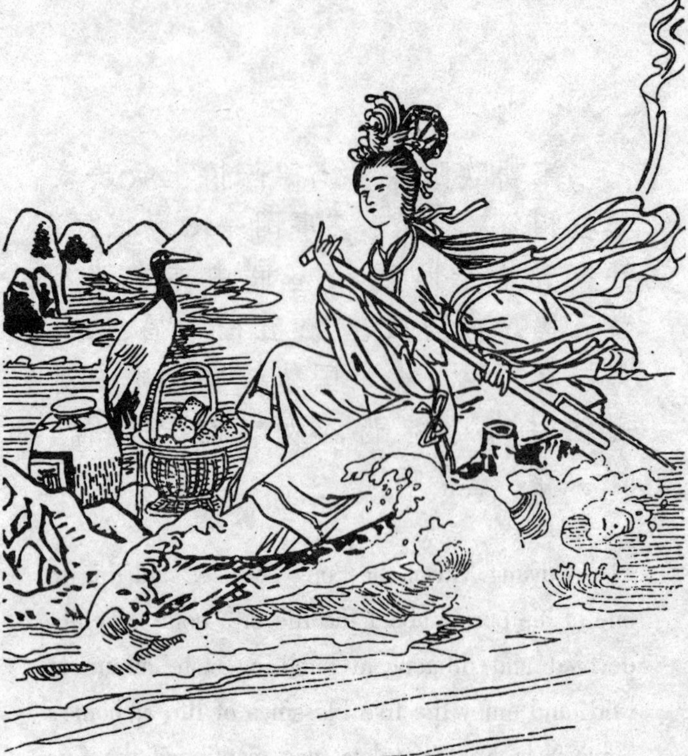

瑶池进酿

Presenting wine to the Queen Mother

《穆天子传》：“乙丑，天子觞西王母于瑶池之上。”瑶池是神话传说中的仙池，为西王母所居仙境，每逢农历三月三，王母在此过寿，宴请群仙。在贺寿的众神中，自然少不了寿仙麻姑，麻姑在绛珠河畔以灵芝酿酒，进献王母。

It is said that every lunar March 3rd, Queen Mother of the West will celebrate her birthday at her celestial dwelling place and invite all the immortals to come. Among these celestial beings, surely the immortal Ma Gu will come after she prepares wine of glossy ganoderma at the celestial riverside. Ma Gu will present the wine to the Queen Mother in her celestial palace.

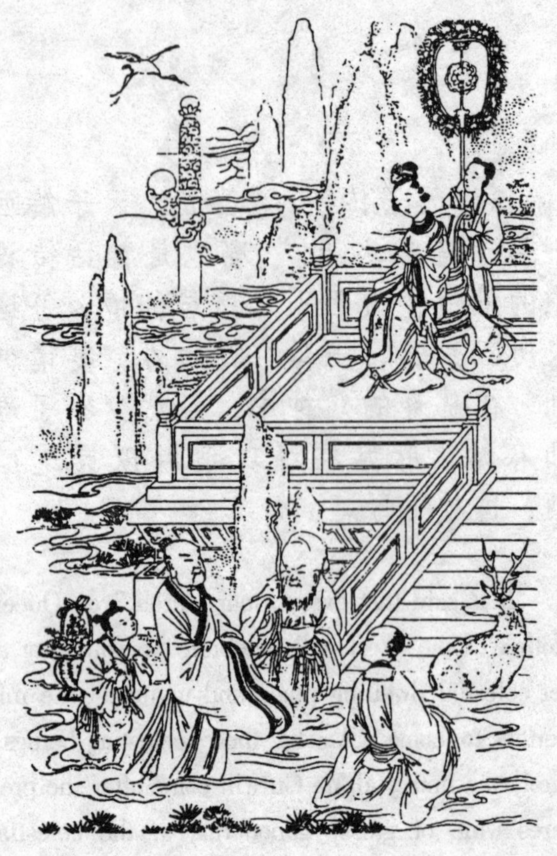

瑶池集庆

Gather to celebrate Queen Mother's birthday

《京都风俗志》："三月三日，相传为西王母蟠桃会之期，东便门内太平宫，俗称蟠桃宫。所居羽士，修建佛寺，自初一至初三庙会，士女拈香，游人甚重。"三月三王母寿宴于瑶池，群仙纷至集会庆贺。寓高朋贵友为长者祝寿。

A book on the customs of old Beijing said that on lunar March 3rd, the day for the peach party arranged by the Queen Mother, a fair would be held in the Peace Palace (also known as Peach Palace) of Beijing for three days. Lots of tourists would gather at the temple and women would burn incenses. At the peach party held in heaven, all immortals would come and congratulate the Queen Mother's birthday. The message is this: friends at prestigious positions come to congratulate the elder's birthday.

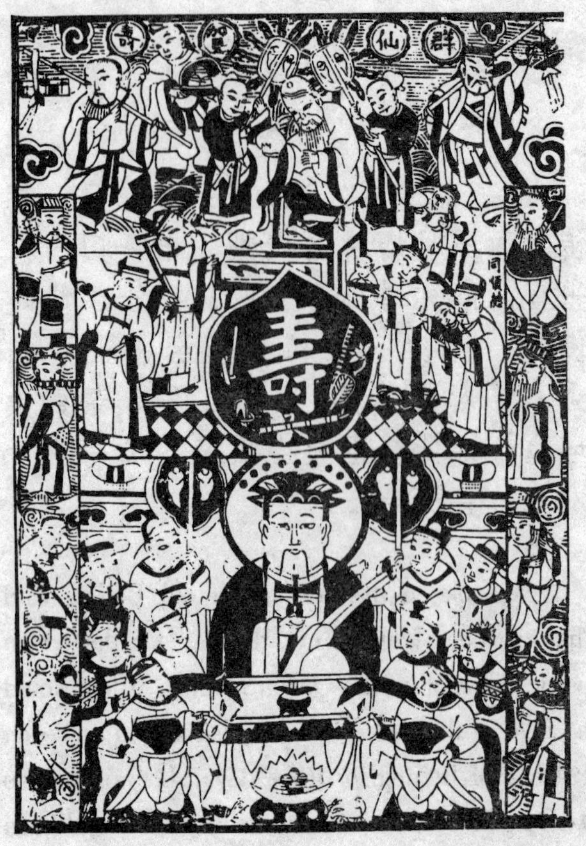

群仙贺寿

All immortals celebrating one's birthday

旧俗对被祝寿人也称“寿星”，老人庆祝生辰称为“庆寿”。中国人自古对“庆寿”非常重视，不仅有亲朋好友“贺寿”，还希望众位神仙“贺寿”，故以吉祥图代之。图中群仙云集，有寿星、有八仙等。群仙贺寿有上寿之福。

In old customs, the central figure of birthday celebrations is the “longevity star”. Chinese has a tradition of grand birthday celebrations: not only should the relatives and good friends be invited, but it would be desirable to have the immortals’ presence as well. Good luck pictures are expressions of such desire. On the picture are the longevity god and the eight immortals, etc. Celestial blessings promise a life of 100 years.

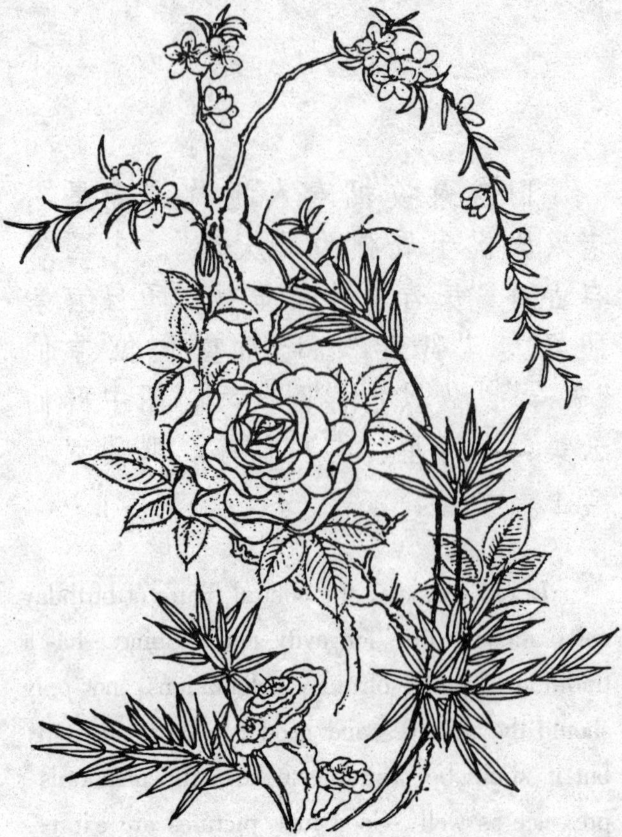

群芳祝寿

Many virtuous people congratulating one's birthday

桃花、月季，花姿绰绰，以代“群芳”。以“竹”谐“祝”，以灵芝喻“寿”。芳指花卉，也指花季，《离骚》：“兰芷变而不芳兮。”芳也喻美名或美德，《晋书》：“后承前训，奉述遗芳。”“群芳祝寿”意为：众多品德美好的人前来祝寿。

Peach blossoms and Chinese roses are beautiful in figure and serve to represent all flowers in the picture. Further, in ancient Chinese writings such as poems by Qu Yuan and some history books, they are the synonyms for good virtues. The picture sends this message: many virtuous people come to congratulate one's birthday.

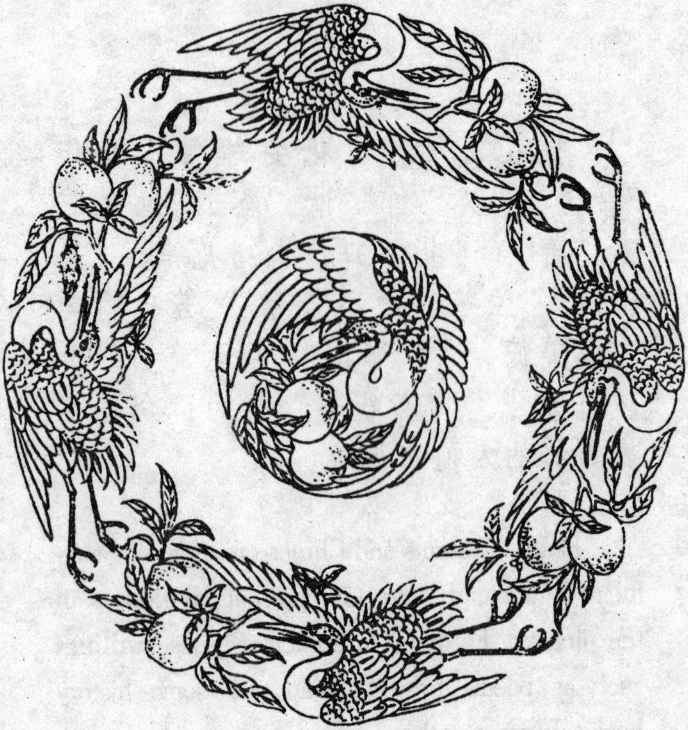

鹤寿千岁

Live to 1,000 *years like the crane and turtle*

《相鹤经》称鹤："寿不可量。"《淮南子》："鹤寿千岁，以极其游。"鹤为长寿仙鹤，在传统观念中鹤与龟同为长寿之王，故世人常以"鹤发童颜"、"龟鹤齐龄"颂长寿之人。旧时寿联有："壮志凤飞逸情云上，灵芳献瑞仙鹤同年。"

Ancient Chinese believed the turtle and crane can live for 1, 000 years or even immeasurably longer. Based on this traditional concept, the turtle and crane are often seen as kings of longevity and many longevity idioms are related to these animals. "To have the crane's hair and a child's face" and "to live as long as the turtle and crane" are two examples. An old couplet goes: "Aspire as the soaring phoenix does and live the long life of a crane".

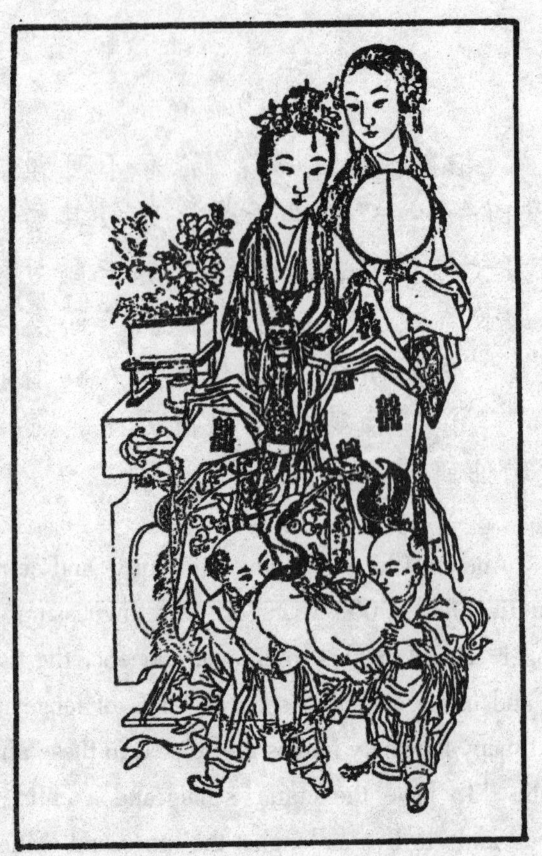

鹤寿之喜

The happiness of longevity

旧时寿幛有："鹤算寿添"、"瑶池桃熟"等。有寿联："蟠桃经三千岁月，鹤算历九十春秋。"两位童子捧桃伴鹤，以示"鹤寿"，并含"贺寿"之喜。图中的妇女带孩子为老人祝寿，这即是老人的福分，又是"孝道"的教育。

Old silk birthday posters had such wordings: Calculate the life of a crane and add years to your own life. Birthday couplets would go: As the flat peaches have grown for 3,000 years, the crane has gone through over 90 seasonal changes. The two kids carry peaches in their hands with a crane next to them, indicating longevity and birthday congratulations. Also in the picture is a woman bringing over her child to congratulate the elder, implying the good fortune of the elder and the importance of filial piety.

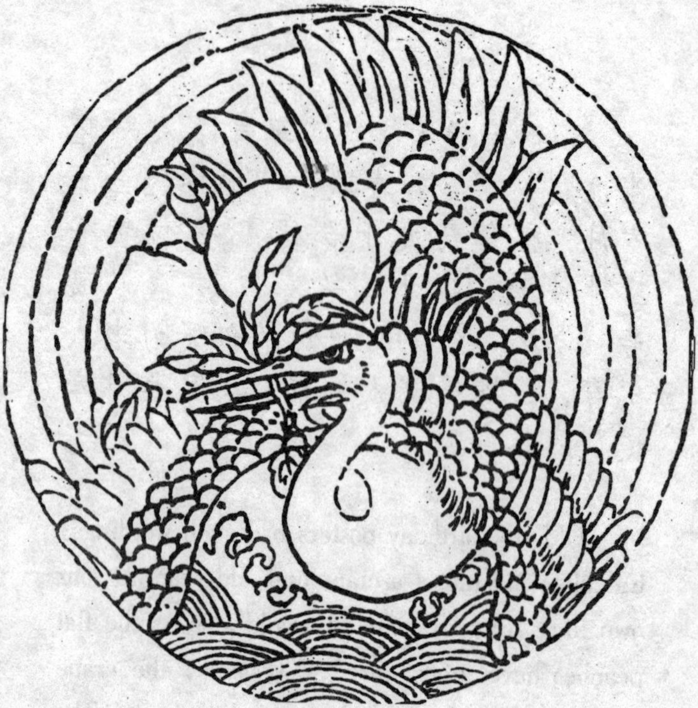

鹤献蟠桃

The crane presents a birthday peach

鹤为长寿仙禽，故常以“鹤寿”、“鹤龄”、“鹤算”等为祝颂人长寿之词。在吉祥图中，鹤与其他长寿之物相配，多表长寿之吉祥。此图鹤衔寿桃，称为“鹤献蟠桃”，为旧时颂寿之语。仙鹤衔仙桃并有水纹组成“团鹤”之形。

Cranes are fairy birds of long life and often quoted in birthday congratulations. In good luck pictures, the crane is matched with other objects related with long life to indicate longevity. The picture here features a crane with a peach in its beak, a common eulogy for birthday celebrations in the past. With the crane surrounded by prints of water waves, the picture forms the shape of a rounded crane.

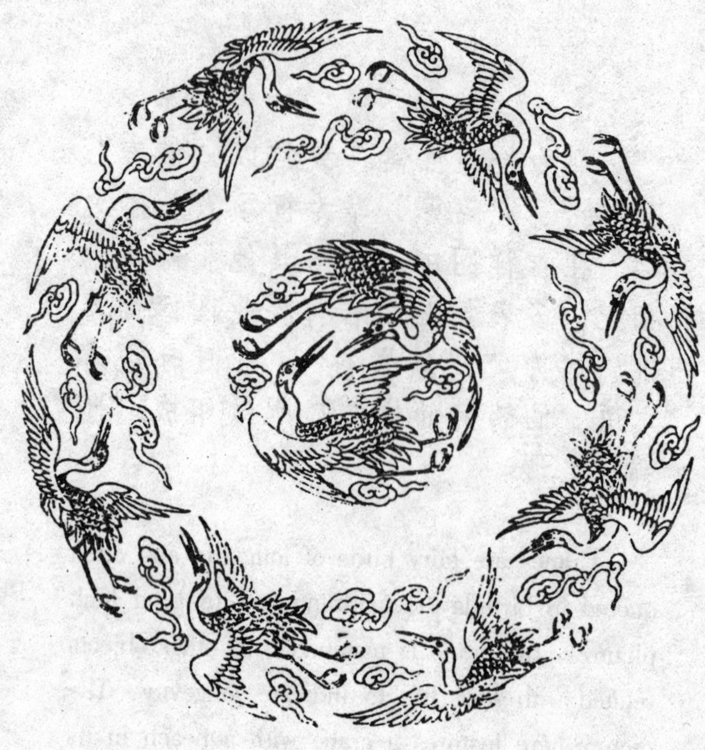

鹤游云天

The crane flies in the sky among the clouds

乾隆皇帝在《三希堂法贴》中，曾为钟繇的书法题字："云鹤游天，群鸿戏海。"《相鹤经》："鹤者阳鸟也，而游于阳。……翔于云，故毛丰而肉疏。"在"群仙仰寿"中，有寿星乘鹤于天，"瑶池集庆"中也有"鹤游云天"。

Emperor Qianlong wrote such inscription for the calligraphy of Zhong Yao: The cranes are flying in the sky and the swan are swimming in the sea. The scene of a crane flying elegantly in the sky is a beautiful and auspicious one. In good luck pictures, the longevity star would ride on a crane. The picture of cranes flying in the sky also appears in other good luck pictures in this book.

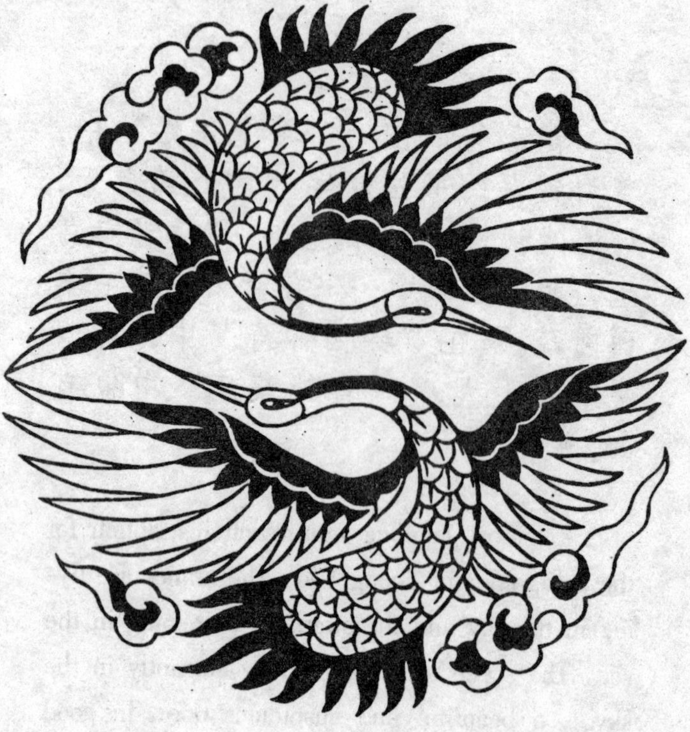

鹤舞祥云

The auspicious scene of dancing cranes

《花镜》：鹤“行必依洲渚，止必集林上。雌雄相随，如道士步斗，履其迹则孕。又雄鸣上风，雌鸣下风，以声交而孕。尝以夜半鸣，声唳九霄，音闻数里。有时雌雄对舞，翱翔上下，宛转跳跃可观。”“鹤舞祥云”为吉兆。

Ancient Chinese had this description of the crane: They walk only on small pieces of land in waters, and gather only on trees in a forest. The male and female cranes follow one another like the Taoist priests taking a walk. Step on their foot prints and women would get pregnant. The male crane would sing in the upper wind and the female in the lower. Their babies are conceived through the interaction of their singing. When they sing at midnight, the sound is so loud that it can be heard several miles away. When they dance to one another, the sight is extremely grand and elegant. Dancing cranes make an auspicious sign.

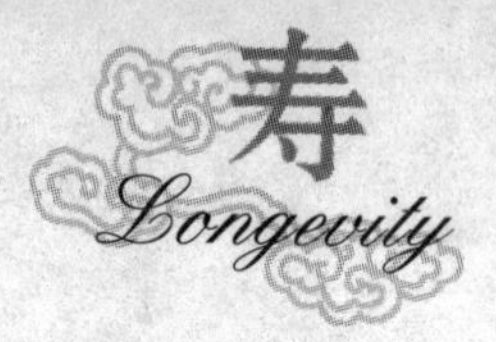

蟠桃千年

Thousands of years of flat peaches

《神农经》："玉桃服之长生不死。若不得早服之，临死服之，其尸毕天地不朽。"桃，有仙桃、寿桃之誉，其中以西王母瑶池所结蟠桃为最，蟠桃三千年一开花，三千年一结实，食一枚可增寿六百岁。故以蟠桃为贺寿之礼。

Flat peaches, according to ancient Chinese records, have the power of turning one immortal. Those who only get to have them at their death bed can leave their bodies unspoiled. The flat peaches grown in the celestial abode of the Queen Mother bloom and bear fruits once every 3,000 years each. One such peach adds to one's life by 600 years. Therefore, flat peaches are common presents for birthday celebrations.

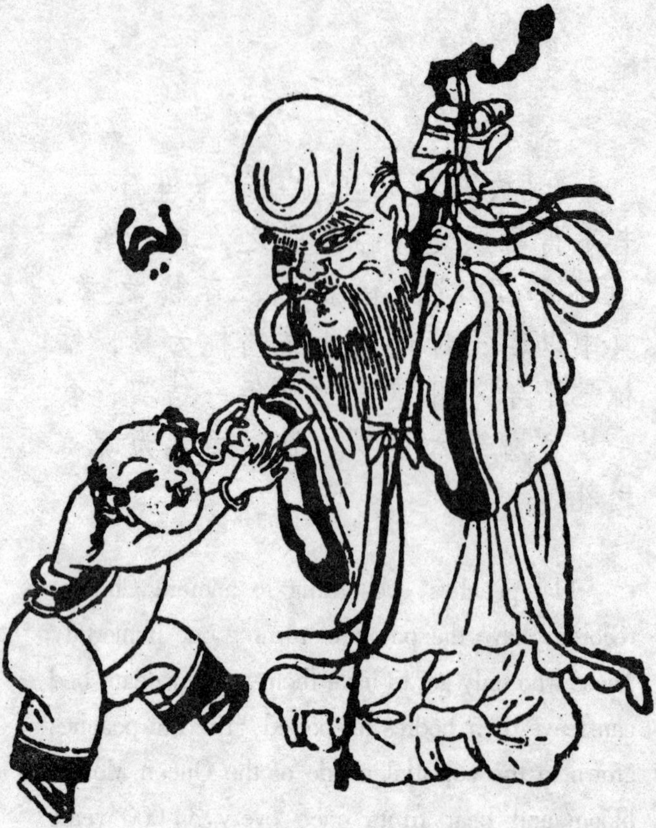

蟠桃上寿

Take flat peaches and live to 100 years

旧时有贺寿联句："玉宇早春六厘东驾，蟠桃上寿一鹤南飞。"《庄子·盗跖》："人，上寿百岁，中寿八十，下寿六十。"王母娘娘有两件宝：一是不死的灵药，一是不老的蟠桃。人受了蟠桃可得上寿，"蟠桃上寿"为祝寿辞。

An old couplet goes: Early in spring, the sun in the east shines on your house; as the crane flies to the south, may flat peaches add your age to 100. Man's life has been categorized by ancient Chinese as supreme longevity of 100 years, medium longevity of 80, and lower longevity of 60. The Queen Mother of the West has two magic objects: a panacea that keeps one alive for always, and peaches that help one stay young. Flat peaches represent 100 years of life.

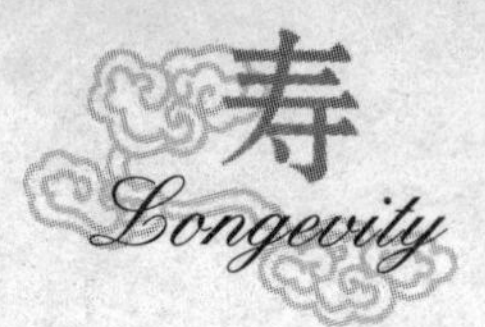

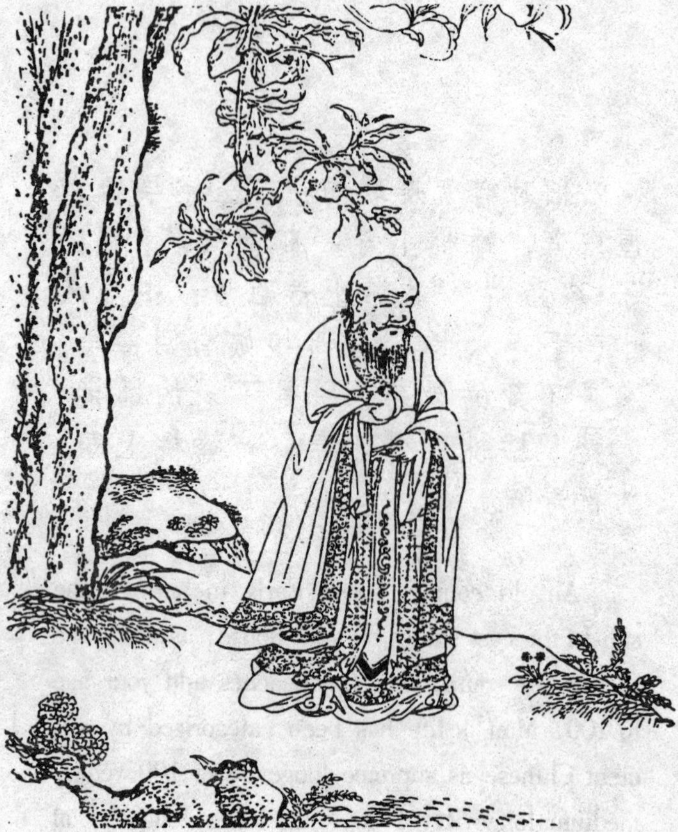

蟠桃献寿

Present flat peaches for birthday celebrations

王母娘娘曾送给汉武帝以蟠桃，东方朔是汉武帝的侍臣，曾到蟠桃园偷桃，成了长生不老之仙。故旧时“蟠桃献寿”图，多画蟠桃树下有一拿桃的仙人，即东方朔，有东方朔献桃则是“千岁蟠桃开寿域，九重春色映霞觞。”

The Queen Mother of the West once offered some flat peaches to Emperor Wu of the Han Dynasty. Dongfang Shuo, a court official of the emperor, went to the peach garden and stole some for himself and turned immortal. Therefore, in the past, an immortal holding a peach under a peach tree often appeared in pictures featuring flat peaches for birthday celebrations. The immortal is Dongfang Shuo and his present adds to the festive air of the celebrations.

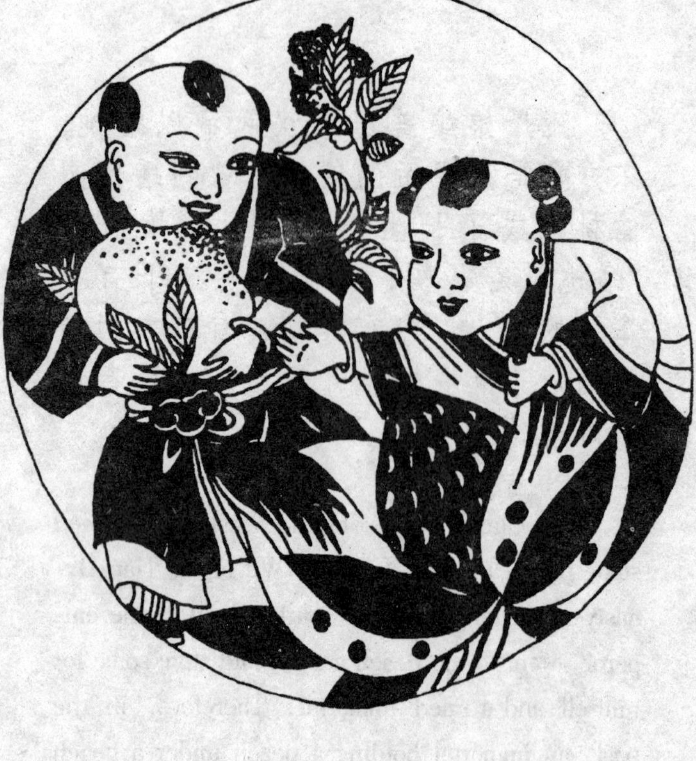

蟠桃献寿

Present flat peaches for birthday celebrations

《都门杂咏》："三月初三春正长，蟠桃宫里看烧香，沿河一带风微起，十丈红尘匝地飏。"描绘了清代北京的蟠桃宫庙会。蟠桃之名源于《海内十洲记》："东海有山名度索山，上有大桃树，蟠屈三千里，曰蟠木。"又称王母桃。

A poem about old Beijing describes the liveliness of the Peach Palace fair of Beijing in the Qing Dynasty: in the spring time of March 3rd, incenses are burnt at the Peach Palace; as a breeze blows up along the river, a vivid picture of the human society is drawn. The name pantao (twining peach trees) comes from such old records: on a mountain called Dusuo in the East Sea grows a large peach tree that twines for over 3000 li. The tree is called the twining tree. The peaches are also called Queen Mother peaches.

图书在版编目（CIP）数据

中华五福吉祥图典.寿 / 黄全信主编；李迎春译.—北京：华语教学出版社，2003.1

ISBN 7 - 80052 - 890 - 1

Ⅰ.中… Ⅱ.①黄… ②李… Ⅲ. 图案 - 中国 - 图集 Ⅳ.J522

中国版本图书馆 CIP 数据核字（2002）第 097611 号

选题策划：单　瑛　英文翻译：李迎春

责任编辑：蔡希勤　封面设计：唐少文

英文编辑：韩　晖　印刷监制：佟汉冬

中华五福吉祥图典—寿

主编　黄全信

*

华语教学出版社出版

（中国北京百万庄路 24 号）

邮政编码 100037

电话: 010-68995871 / 68326333

传真: 010-68326333

电子信箱: hyjx @263.net

北京通州次渠印刷厂印刷

中国国际图书贸易总公司海外发行

（中国北京车公庄西路 35 号）

北京邮政信箱第 399 号　邮政编码 100044

新华书店国内发行

2003 年（32 开）第一版

（汉英）

ISBN 7-80052-890 -1 / H · 1426（外）

9－CE－3527P

定价：26.00 元

Printed in China